MEDICAL MASTERCLASS

Nephrology

Disclaimer

Although every effort has been made to ensure that drug doses and other information are presented accurately in this publication, the ultimate responsibility rests with the prescribing physician. Neither the publishers nor the authors can be held responsible for any consequences arising from the use of information contained herein. Any product mentioned in this publication should be used in accordance with the prescribing information prepared by the manufacturers.

The information presented in this publication reflects the opinions of its contributors and should not be taken to represent the policy and views of the Royal College of Physicians of London, unless this is specifically stated.

Every effort has been made by the contributors to contact holders of copyright to obtain permission to reproduce copyright material. However, if any have been inadvertently overlooked, the publisher will be pleased to make the necessary arrangements at the first opportunity.

Medical Masterclass

EDITOR-IN-CHIEF

John D. Firth DM FRCP

Consultant Physician and Nephrologist

Addenbrooke's Hospital

Cambridge

Nephrology

EDITOR

Patrick H. Maxwell MRCP MA MBBS DPhil

Lecturer and Honorary Consultant

University of Oxford

Oxford

Blackwell Science

© 2001 Royal College of Physicians of
London, 11 St Andrews Place, London
NW1 4LE,
Registered Charity No. 210508

Published by:
Blackwell Science Ltd
Editorial Offices:
Osney Mead, Oxford OX2 0EL
25 John Street, London WC1N 2BS
23 Ainslie Place, Edinburgh EH3 6AJ
350 Main Street, Malden
    MA 02148-5018, USA
54 University Street, Carlton
    Victoria 3053, Australia
10, rue Casimir Delavigne
    75006 Paris, France

Other Editorial Offices:
Blackwell Wissenschafts-Verlag GmbH
Kurfürstendamm 57
10707 Berlin, Germany

Blackwell Science KK
MG Kodenmacho Building
7–10 Kodenmacho Nihombashi
Chuo-ku, Tokyo 104, Japan

Iowa State University Press
A Blackwell Science Company
2121 S. State Avenue
Ames, Iowa 50014-8300, USA

First published 2001

Set by Graphicraft Limited, Hong Kong
Printed and bound in Italy by Rotolito
Lombarda SpA, Milan

Catalogue records for this title are available
from the British Library and the Library of
Congress

ISBN 0-632-05871-4 (this book)
    0-632-05567-7 (set)

Commissioning Editors: Mike Stein and
    Rachel Robson
Project Manager (RCP): Filipa Maia
Editorial Assistant (RCP): Katherine Bowker
Production: Charlie Hamlyn and Jonathan
    Rowley
Layout and Cover Design: Chris Stone

DISTRIBUTORS

Marston Book Services Ltd
PO Box 269
Abingdon, Oxon OX14 4YN
(Orders: Tel: 01235 465500
        Fax: 01235 465555)

USA
Blackwell Science, Inc.
Commerce Place
350 Main Street
Malden, MA 02148-5018
(Orders: Tel: 800 759 6102
        781 388 8250
    Fax: 781 388 8255)

Canada
Login Brothers Book Company
324 Saulteaux Crescent
Winnipeg, Manitoba R3J 3T2
(Orders: Tel: 204 837 2987)

Australia
Blackwell Science Pty Ltd
54 University Street
Carlton, Victoria 3053
(Orders: Tel: 3 9347 0300
        Fax: 3 9347 5001)

For further information on
Blackwell Science, visit our website:
www.blackwell-science.com

Contents

List of contributors

Nick C. Fluck MBBS BSc MRCP DPhil
Consultant in Nephrology and General Medicine
Aberdeen Royal Infirmary
Aberdeen

Philip Kalra MA MB BChir FRCP MD
Consultant and Honorary University Lecturer
Department of Nephrology
Hope Hospital
Salford

Patrick H. Maxwell MRCP MA MBBS DPhil
Lecturer and Honorary Consultant
University of Oxford
Oxford

Chris A. O'Callaghan BA BM BCh MA MRCP DPhil
Medical Research Council Clinical Scientist
John Radcliffe Hospital
Oxford

Foreword

Medical Masterclass is the most innovative and important educational development from the Royal College of Physicians in the last 100 years. Throughout our 480-year history we have pioneered and supported high-quality medicine, and while *Medical Masterclass* continues that tradition, it also represents a quantum leap for the College as it moves into the 21st century.

The effort that the College has put in to improve the Membership Examination, which started 150 years ago and is now run by all three UK Royal Colleges of Physicians, will now be matched by its attention to basic learning in general medicine—the grounding and preparation for the exam.

Teaching and learning for the exam have changed little over the past 50 years, relying on local courses, word-based teaching and commercial courses. *Medical Masterclass* is a completely new approach for those wishing to practise high-quality medicine. It is an imaginative multimedia programme with paper and CD modules covering the major areas of medicine, supported by a website which will provide summaries and links to the latest articles and guidelines, and self-assessment questionnaires with feedback. Its focus is on self-learning, self-assessment and dealing with realistic clinical problems—not just force-feeding facts. The series of interactive case studies on which the modules are based entail making diagnostic and treatment decisions, closely mimicking the situations found in the admission suite or outpatient clinic.

Medical Masterclass has been produced by the RCP's Education Department together with Blackwell Science. It represents a formidable amount of work by Dr John Firth and his team of authors and editors and is set to be the jewel in our crown. It also signals very clearly our intention to lead in the field of learning and to be supportive to our future members. I anticipate the package will also be invaluable for continued learning by our specialist registrars and consultants as part of continuing professional development.

I congratulate our colleagues for this superb product and commend it to you without reservation.

Professor Sir George Alberti
President of the Royal College of Physicians, London

Preface

Medical Masterclass comprises twelve paper-based modules, two CD-ROMs and a companion website. Its aim is to help doctors in their first few years of training to improve their medical skills and knowledge.

The twelve paper-based modules are divided as follows: two cover the scientific background to medicine, one is devoted to general clinical issues, one to emergency medicine and practical procedures, and eight cover the range of medical specialities. Medicine is often fairly straightforward when the diagnosis is clear, but patients rarely come to their doctor and say 'I've got Hodgkin's disease': they have lumps. The core material of each of the clinical specialities is defined by case presentations in the first part of each module: how do you approach the man who has lumps? Structured concise notes on specific diseases follow later. All practising doctors know that medicine is much more than knowing lots of facts about diseases: how do you tell someone they've got cancer? How do you decide when to stop treatment? Most medical texts say little about these issues: *Medical Masterclass* does not avoid them, nor does it talk in vague and abstract terms.

The two CD-ROMs each contain 30 interactive cases requiring diagnosis and treatment. The format is remarkably close to real life: you see the patient and are told the story; you have to decide how to investigate and treat; but you can't see all the results before you start to make decisions!

The companion website, which will be regularly updated, includes literature and guideline updates and review, and self-assessment questions. How much do you know, and are you improving? You will see how your score compares with your previous attempts, and also how your performance compares with others who have logged on to the site.

The *Medical Masterclass* is produced by the Education Department of the Royal College of Physicians of London and published by Blackwell Science. It is not a crammer for the MRCP exam and not written by those who set the exam. However, I have no doubt that someone putting effort into learning through the *Medical Masterclass* would be in a strong position to impress the examiners, although I am afraid that success—like much else in medicine and in life—cannot be guaranteed.

John Firth
Editor-in-Chief

Acknowledgements

Medical Masterclass has been produced by a team. The names of those who have written and edited material are clearly indicated elsewhere, but without the efforts of many other people *Medical Masterclass* would not exist at all. These include Professor Lesley Rees and Mrs Winnie Wade from the Education Department of the Royal College of Physicians of London, who initiated the project; Dr Mike Stein and Dr Andy Robinson from Medschool.com and Blackwell Science respectively, who have enthusiastically supported it from the beginning; and Ms Filipa Maia and Ms Katherine Bowker, who have run the office with splendid efficiency and induced authors and editors to perform to a schedule rarely achieved. I and the whole of the team of editors and authors are immensely grateful to all of these people for the energy that they have poured into *Medical Masterclass* in various ways.

John Firth
Editor-in-Chief

Key features

We have created a range of icon boxes to help you identify key information and to make learning easier and more enjoyable. Here is a brief explanation:

 Clinical pointer

This icon highlights important information to be noted.

 Further information

This icon indicates the source of further information and reference.

 Hints

This icon highlights useful hints, tips and mnemonics.

 Key points

This icon is used to highlight points of particular importance.

 Quote

This icon indicates useful or interesting citations from notable individuals, including well-known physicians.

 Think about

This icon indicates what the reader should reflect on after having read a passage from the text.

 Warning/Hazard

This icon is used to indicate common or important drug interactions, pitfalls of practical procedures, or when to take symptoms or signs particularly seriously.

Nephrology

AUTHORS:
**N. Fluck, P.A. Kalra, P.H. Maxwell,
C.A. O'Callaghan**

EDITOR:
P.H. Maxwell

EDITOR-IN-CHIEF:
J.D. Firth

1 Clinical presentations

1.1 Routine medical shows dipstick haematuria

Case history

A 43-year-old airline pilot is found to have a positive urine dipstick test for blood at an insurance medical. There is also a trace of protein. He has no symptoms. His blood pressure is 142/94 mmHg.

Clinical approach

Everyone has some red blood cells in their urine. Urine dipstick tests are very sensitive and are capable of detecting concentrations of red blood cells at the upper limit of the normal range for red cell excretion. Between 2.5% and 13% of men have positive urine dipstick tests for blood, which in most cases is not associated with significant disease. Recognized causes of haematuria are shown in Table 1.

The clinical approach depends on the age of the patient (Fig. 1):
• In a young person, haematuria is usually glomerular in origin (most frequently as a result of IgA nephropathy) and tumours are rare.
• In an elderly patient, tumours within the kidney or urinary tract are an important cause.
• Stones can cause haematuria at any age.

Evaluation of isolated microscopic haematuria is dependent on patient age:
• Above 45: IVU (intravenous urogram) or urinary tract ultrasound and plain film encompassing kidneys, ureter and bladder (KUB); cystoscopy
• Below 45: more likely to be glomerular, so initial assessment nephrological.

Table 1 Differential diagnosis of haematuria.

Source of bleeding	Common and important	Other causes
Kidney	Glomerulonephritis— especially IgA nephropathy Adult polycystic kidney disease Tumours	Thin membrane disease —benign familial haematuria Interstitial nephritis Papillary necrosis Alport's syndrome Loin pain haematuria syndrome
Urinary tract/bladder	Tumours Prostatic disease—benign or malignant Urinary stones	

Also consider: trauma; gynaecological bleeding.

History of the presenting problem

Background history

Although the patient is currently asymptomatic, ask carefully about the symptoms described below.

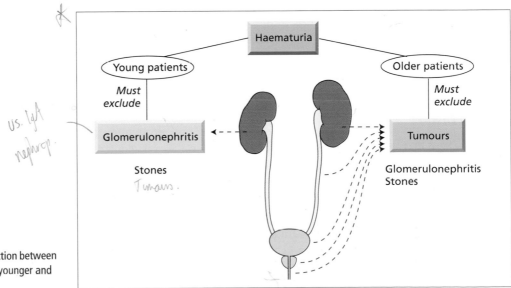

Fig. 1 This figure shows the distinction between the investigation of haematuria in younger and older patients.

Frank haematuria

If present, ask whether blood was at the start (from the urethra or prostate) or the end of the stream (from the bladder). Blood clots are unusual with glomerular bleeding.

Episodes of frank haematuria, especially at the same time or just after a mild upper respiratory tract infection, are consistent with IgA nephropathy. Frank haematuria followed by persistent microscopic haematuria strongly suggests IgA nephropathy.

Frank haematuria also occurs with stones and tumours.

Pain

Ask about previous pain in the loin, the abdomen, the groin and the external genitalia.
• Pain is consistent with stones or tumours, polycystic kidney disease, loin pain haematuria syndrome, renal infection or infarction.
• Painless haematuria is consistent with tumours, glomerulonephritis, interstitial nephritis or a bleeding disorder.

General history

Enquire about the following:
• Recent trauma or heavy exercise, which can cause dipstick haematuria
• Joint pains or skin rashes, suggesting a multi-system disorder such as systemic vasculitis
• A sore throat or other recent infection, raising the possibility of a postinfective glomerulonephritis.

Urinary symptoms

Ask about the following:
• Dysuria and increased urinary frequency, which suggest acute infection
• Symptoms of a poor urinary stream such as hesitancy, poor flow and dribbling; these are consistent with prostatic or bladder pathology
• Previous passage of stones, grit or gravel.

Family history

Ask about hereditary renal conditions, especially polycystic kidney disease and Alport's syndrome (which also causes hearing problems).

Note that other inherited conditions can cause haematuria:
• In sickle cell disease, sickling can damage and occlude vessels, causing medullary ischaemia and bleeding
• Many patients with haemophilia or von Willebrand's disease experience microscopic or frank haematuria.

Social history

Ask about travel to areas where *Schistosoma haematobium* is prevalent because infection can cause urinary tract granuloma and tumour formation.

Drug history

Ask specifically about analgesics which can cause papillary necrosis and therefore haematuria. Note that this does not happen with occasional use of analgesics and has become much less common since phenacetin was withdrawn from compound analgesic preparations. The typical story would be of chronic headache or back pain, with the patient consuming 10–20 or more analgesic tablets per day for many years.

Examination

The following are important:
• Check the blood pressure
• Look for signs of multi-system diseases (such as skin or joint lesions)
• Look for signs of infection consistent with an infection-related glomerulonephritis
• Check for renal enlargement, possibly caused by tumours or polycystic kidney disease, and also for renal tenderness
• Examine the optic fundus
• Examine the pelvis and external genitalia, and the prostate in men
• Consider gynaecological examination, if there is suspicion of a pelvic tumour extending into the urinary system in women.

 Always check the blood pressure in anyone with suspected renal disease.

Approach to investigations and management

Investigation

Urinalysis and microscopy

Proteinuria combined with haematuria suggests renal disease: glomerulonephritis or interstitial nephritis (less likely). If there is dipstick proteinuria, as in this man, then quantify this with a 24-h collection or by measuring the protein/creatinine ratio. In this patient a 24-h collection contained 0.8 g protein.

Dysmorphic red cells on microscopy suggest glomerular bleeding, but morphological changes can occur as artefacts after collection of the sample; the distinction of dysmorphic cells (from the kidney) from non-dysmorphic cells (from the urinary drainage system) requires special expertise and is not a routine or reliable test in most centres.

 Red blood cell casts indicate active glomerular inflammation.

Renal function

Check plasma urea and creatinine. Calculate the predicted glomerular filtration rate (GFR) based on sex, age and weight (see Section 3.2, pp. 107–108). Remember that there can be a substantial fall in GFR before serum creatinine rises out of the normal range.

If renal function is normal, blood pressure is normal and there is no significant proteinuria, significant medical renal pathology is very unlikely.

This patient's plasma creatinine was 190 μmol/L, giving a predicted GFR of 42 mL/min, which is a very substantial reduction for a man of this age.

Imaging

Image the renal tract to exclude stones and assess renal size and anatomy. The best way of doing this is to order both:
• Plain radiograph (KUB or kidneys, ureter, bladder): looking for stones
• Ultrasonography of the urinary tract: to measure renal size (preferably length of each kidney in centimetres: not normal or small), look for renal masses and carefully examine the bladder wall.

Other imaging approaches can be useful in some cases:
• IVU: to determine whether small calcific lesions are urinary stones, and whether stones are causing obstruction
• Computed tomography (CT): characterize any abnormality seen on ultrasonography.

In this patient, renal ultrasonography showed normal-size kidneys (right 11 cm, left 11.5 cm in length).

Urological investigation

In an older person, arrange cystoscopy to look for a tumour in the lower urinary tract.

Renal biopsy

Given the borderline hypertension, proteinuria and impaired renal function, glomerular disease was considered likely and renal biopsy was performed to make a precise diagnosis; this showed IgA nephropathy.

Management

Management of IgA nephropathy remains controversial (see Section 2.3, p. 75) and no specific therapy has achieved acceptance. Measures to prevent progressive renal damage should be considered, as in other patients with significant renal disease (see Section 2.1, pp. 48–61). Particularly important is antihypertensive treatment: if the single blood pressure recorded in this patient is confirmed by other readings, then an angiotensin-converting enzyme (ACE) inhibitor would be started.

 Blood pressure control slows the rate of renal deterioration in chronic renal impairment. ACE inhibitors are particularly effective.

Communication points

The patient may feel more comfortable with or without discussion of the diagnosis and prognosis (see Section 2.3, pp. 72–79). The extent of tubulointerstitial disease on the biopsy and the amount of proteinuria are both important prognostic indicators in IgA nephropathy.

It is important to consider that the diagnosis may adversely affect the patient's ability to obtain life insurance and may have implications for their employment.

 Kincaid-Smith P. Treatment of mesangial immunoglobulin A glomerulonephritis. *Semin Nephrol* 1999; 19: 166–172. Sinniah R, Pwee HS, Lim CH. Glomerular lesions in asymptomatic microscopic haematuria discovered on routine medical examination. *Clin Nephrol* 1976; 5: 216–228.

1.2 Pregnancy with renal disease

Case history

A previously healthy 26-year-old woman booked with her GP for her first pregnancy check. Routine urinary dipstick analysis identified 2+ proteinuria. Mid-stream urine (MSU) was negative and a subsequent 24-h urine collection gave 1.2 g protein/24 h. She is now 16 weeks pregnant; urea is 6 mmol/L and creatinine 109 μmol/L.

Clinical approach

Before seeing the patient, you ask the GP to arrange renal ultrasonography, which shows bilateral scars and establishes the diagnosis of reflux nephropathy. You will need to assess the patient's current clinical state and consider other differential diagnoses of proteinuria. Clearly, the patient is going to be worried. She has suddenly learned that she has a kidney problem and will have pressing questions:
• Will I be all right?

- Will the baby survive and be healthy?
- Will I develop kidney failure?

Before seeing the patient, make sure that you have accurate information about renal impairment and pregnancy. You will need to liaise closely with obstetric colleagues to ensure a consistent approach.

This patient has presented early in pregnancy, but in those who present later it can be difficult to distinguish proteinuria and hypertension related to pre-eclampsia from intrinsic renal disease. It may only be possible to tell whether there is intrinsic renal disease after the end of the pregnancy.

History of the presenting problem

Symptoms of reflux nephropathy include nocturnal enuresis, recurrent urinary tract infections and loin pain but there may be no symptoms at all.

Relevant past history

There may be a childhood history suggestive of vesicoureteric reflux (see Section 2.4, p. 85).

Family history

Many cases of vesicoureteric reflux have a genetic component. Has anyone else in the family had similar problems? (See Section 2.4, p. 85.)

Examination

Record:
- Blood pressure (in pregnancy, Korotkoff phase V may not occur and the diastolic can be taken when the sound becomes muffled—Korotkoff IV)
- Weight
- Urinary dipstick findings
- Oedema.

Approach to investigations and management

Investigations

Baseline tests should include:
- Creatinine, electrolytes and liver function tests
- Uric acid (useful in monitoring pre-eclampsia)
- Full blood count (FBC)
- 24-h urine for protein and creatinine clearance
- Urine culture.

Measuring renal function and blood pressure in pregnancy

Normal changes in cardiovascular physiology during preg-

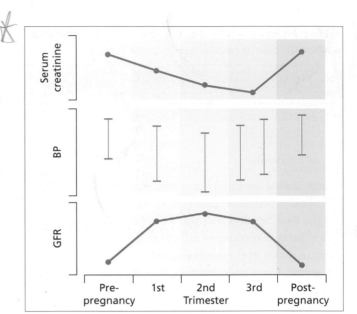

Fig. 2 Schematic diagram illustrating the changes in blood pressure, serum creatinine and glomerular filtration rate during pregnancy.

nancy lead to changes in both blood pressure and excretory renal function (Fig. 2). This means that evaluation of blood pressure, serum creatinine and 24-h creatinine clearance results requires consideration of the stage of pregnancy.

Our patient is in the second trimester, at which time the BP should reach its nadir and average serum creatinine falls from 73 to 51 μmol as a result of a 50% increase in GFR. Thus, our patient has significantly impaired renal function, even though the serum creatinine (109 μmol/L) is within the 'normal' range (up to 125 μmol/L).

Management

This is based on an understanding of the issues involved.

Risks to the mother and baby

Pre-existing renal disease is associated with increased maternal and fetal complications. There appears to be a threshold value of creatinine above which there is a sharp increase in problems. Changes in the slope of the reciprocal creatinine suggest that women with a creatinine greater than 125 μmol/L have a significant risk of accelerated decline. This is often irreversible and may ultimately lead to end-stage renal failure and dialysis (Table 2).

Specific data in patients with reflux nephropathy suggest that the prognosis in this group may be worse than in other renal disease (Table 3). Furthermore, in the small number of patients reported with reflux and a creatinine greater than 200 μmol/L, rapid decline in function with dialysis within 2 years is common.

Hypertension in these patients is of particular importance. If present, the risk of renal deterioration increases about five-fold, and there are also risks to the baby, with

Table 2 Pregnancy-related problems in women with pre-existing renal disease.

Impairment of renal function pre-pregnancy or 1st trimester	Maternal complications	Fetal loss
Mild (Creatinine <125 μmol/L)	Common (≈25%)	Rare (<5%)
Moderate (Creatinine 125–250 μmol/L)	Very common (≈50%)	Uncommon (<10%)
Severe (Creatinine >250 μmol/L)	Nearly all (≈90%)	Very common (≈50%)

Table 3 Pregnancy-related problems in women with reflux nephropathy [2].

Impairment of renal function	Deterioration in renal function (%)	Pre-eclampsia (%)	Fetal loss (%)
Mild (Creatinine <110 μmol/L)	2	13	8
Moderate (Creatinine >110 μmol/L)	18	30	18

double the rate of pre-term delivery and a six-fold increase in intrauterine growth retardation.

 Reflux nephropathy has a strong genetic component. The baby will need evaluation by a paediatrician after birth.

Management of the mother

The obstetric team will take primary responsibility for managing the pregnancy. She should be seen every 2 weeks until 32 weeks, and then weekly. Attention should be paid to the following:
• Urinary tract infections: these are common in reflux nephropathy and in pregnancy, but may be asymptomatic. Positive MSUs should be treated. Recurrent infections warrant prophylactic antibiotics.
• Hypertension: this should be monitored carefully and treated vigorously. Suitable agents include α-methyldopa, labetalol, nifedipine and hydralazine.
• Fetal surveillance.
• Timing of delivery: this is primarily an obstetric decision; delivery is usually appropriate if maternal problems are escalating or there is fetal distress.

COMMUNICATION

Advise this patient of the following:
• The pregnancy should be successful but requires close monitoring by her obstetric team
• She will probably need BP treatment as there is an increased risk of pre-eclampsia
• There may be some loss of kidney function and a small chance of serious deterioration

• The baby has a higher chance of being smaller than usual and needing to be delivered pre-term
• After the birth, her baby will need investigation to rule out a similar kidney condition.

 To give useful advice about possible risks and likely outcomes, you need precise knowledge. A vague idea is unlikely to be good enough.

Management of the child

Fetal ultrasonography is possible. The renal tract can usually be visualized after 20 weeks: if abnormal this will prompt early postnatal investigations.

A micturating cystourethrogram is the standard screening investigation used in young children and babies. Other radiological investigations may provide complimentary information:
• Renal ultrasonography is non-invasive and can detect structural abnormalities and upper tract dilatation
• Isotope imaging techniques using agents such as ^{99m}Tc-dimercaptosuccinic acid (DMSA) can identify cortical scars.

Long-term antibiotic prophylaxis is the usual initial treatment.

El-Khatib M, Packham DK, Becker GJ, Kincaid-Smith P. Pregnancy-related complications in women with reflux nephropathy. *Clin Nephrol* 1994; 41: 50–54.
Hou S. Pregnancy in chronic renal insufficiency and end-stage renal disease. *Am J Kid Disease* 1999; 33: 235–253.
Woolf AS. Primary vesicoureteric reflux and associated nephropathies. In: *Horizons in Medicine*, No. 12 (Pusey C, ed.) London: Royal College of Physicians of London, 1999: 325–333.

1.3 A swollen young woman

Case history

A 22-year-old female teacher presents with a 1-week history of feeling tired, slightly breathless and swelling up. She has peripheral oedema. Dipstick urinalysis by her GP reveals 4+ proteinuria with no haematuria.

Clinical approach

There are many causes of breathlessness and ankle swelling in a young woman, including cardiopulmonary conditions such as cardiomyopathy and primary pulmonary

Table 4 Causes of the nephrotic syndrome.

Common	Rare
Primary glomerular disease	Constrictive pericarditis
Minimal change nephropathy	Sickle cell disease
Focal segmental glomerulosclerosis	Hereditary renal disease
Membranous nephropathy	(e.g. 'Finnish type' nephrotic
IgA nephropathy	syndrome, Familial
IgA nephropathy	Mediterranean Fever)
Mesangiocapillary (or membranoproliferative glomerulonephritis)	Allergies (e.eg. bee sting,
Diffuse proliferative glomerulonephritis (or acute endocapillary	penicillin)
glomerulonephritis)	Accelerated hypertension
Antiglomerular basement disease (or Goodpasture's disease)	Toxins (e.g. petroleum-based
Crescent glomerulonephritis (or rapidly progressive	hydro-carbons, poison ivy
glomerulonephritis, focal necrotizing glomerulonephritis or renal	or oak)
microscopic polyangiitis)	Alport's syndrome
	glomerulonephritis
Secondary glomerular disease	
Diabetes mellitus	
Myeloma	
Amyloidosis	
Pre-eclampsia	
Drugs (e.g. gold, penicillamine, captropril, NSAIDs)	
Infections (e.g. malaria, hepatitis B, leprosy)	
Connective tissue disease (e.g. SLE)	
Malignancy (e.g. lymphoma, carcinoma, CLL)	

hypertension. Here the amount of protein on urinalysis, a simple bedside test, suggests nephrotic syndrome [1].

It is important to do the following:
- Confirm the nephrotic syndrome by measurement of serum albumin (should be low: <35 g/L) and 24-h urinary protein excretion (should be high: >3 g)
- Assess whether there is renal impairment
- Identify the precise underlying glomerular disease by renal biopsy.

The many causes of the nephrotic syndrome are shown in Table 4—which of these has the patient got? Symptomatic treatment with diuretics may clear the oedema, but specific therapy may be indicated by the renal biopsy findings and/or disease associations.

History of the presenting problem

In this case, primary glomerular disease is the most likely cause of the nephrotic syndrome. However, a thorough clinical history should be taken to look for clues to any of the causes listed in Table 4. Ask questions related to the following.

The nephrotic state

- Oedema: for how long has the patient noticed this? Did it come on suddenly? How much has her weight changed? Rapid onset of severe oedema is more common in minimal change nephrotic syndrome.
- Change in weight (if known) can be used as an indication of how much salt and water has been retained.

- Urine: has the patient noticed a change? Heavy proteinuria causes frothy urine and this can help to date the onset of problems.
- The nephrotic syndrome can be complicated by venous thromboembolism; has one leg been more swollen than the other? Has her breathing been OK? Has she had any chest pain or haemoptysis?

Causes of the nephrotic syndrome

- Nephrotic syndrome may be secondary to many other conditions (Table 4): in a young woman, systemic lupus erythematosus (SLE) is an important consideration. Is there anything in the history to suggest this? (See Section 1.9, pp. 28–31; see *Rheumatology and clinical immunology*, Sections 1.11, 1.12 and 2.4.1.)
- Drugs: a range of over-the-counter and prescribed medications can cause the nephrotic syndrome, as can intravenous drug abuse.
- Minimal change nephrotic syndrome often relapses and remits. Has she ever had this problem before?
- Alport's syndrome (see Section 2.8.2, p. 104) can be associated with nephrotic-range proteinuria, and familial forms of other glomerulonephritides are recognized (e.g. focal segmental glomerulosclerosis).

Examination

Assess the severity of the nephrotic state. In particular note the following:

• Weigh the patient and compare with previous values (if known).
• Blood pressure: despite oedema there may be intravascular fluid depletion (hypovolaemia). Look for postural hypotension. Some forms of renal disease will be associated with hypertension, but this is rare with minimal change disease.
• Examine for pleural effusions and ascites.
• Examine the oedema: this may be associated with skin breakdown and cellulitis. Remember that any detectable oedema implies at least a 2-L increase in extracellular fluid, and that in the nephrotic syndrome there is often a 10-L increase in extracellular fluid volume.
• Look for evidence of other conditions listed in Table 4, SLE in particular in this case.
• Is there any clinical evidence of deep vein thrombosis or pulmonary embolism? (See *Cardiology*, Section 1.9.)

Postural hypotension is the best physical sign in hypovolaemia.

Approach to investigations and management

Investigations

Bedside tests

Examine the urine—repeat dipstick urinalysis and perform microscopy of the spun deposit. Microscopic haematuria can occur in minimal change nephrotic syndrome, but (particularly if heavy) suggests another diagnosis. Red cell casts would point to active glomerular inflammation.

Blood biochemistry

Check renal and liver function and serum cholesterol:
• Serum creatinine: this may be high in some types of the nephrotic syndrome, e.g. membranous glomerulonephritis, or in elderly patients with minimal change glomerulonephritis. Our patient had a serum creatinine of 65 µmol/L.
• Serum albumin: this is low in the nephrotic syndrome, especially so in less well-nourished patients (e.g. elderly), those with systemic disease (hepatic albumin synthesis reduced) and in those with gross proteinuria (e.g. >10 g/24 h).
• Cholesterol: this will be elevated, and may be very high (>10 mmol/L) when proteinuria is gross.

24-h urine collection

Measure 24-h urinary protein excretion and creatinine clearance. In this case this confirms nephrotic range proteinuria (>3 g/24 h) and creatinine clearance—calculated as an estimate of GFR (see Section 3.2, pp. 107–108)—is 93 mL/min.

Many patients find it difficult to perform 24-h urine collections, in which case proteinuria can be estimated from a spot urine sample, factoring the concentration of albumin in the specimen by that of creatinine. In a normal adult the value of the albumin/creatinine ratio (ACR) is less than 21 mg albumin/mmol creatinine; those with nephrotic range proteinuria will have a value >360 mg/mmol.

The degree of selectivity of proteinuria is not sufficiently useful to be routinely measured in adult practice, but highly selective proteinuria (i.e. mainly albumin) suggests minimal change glomerulonephritis.

Other blood tests

Check the following:
• Inflammatory markers: C-reactive protein (CRP) and erythrocyte sedimentation rate (ESR)
• Evidence of SLE: antinuclear factor (ANF), double-stranded DNA (dsDNA) and further specific tests if indicated
• Serum complement levels: C3 and/or C4 may be depressed in some forms of glomerulonephritis, particularly SLE
• Immunoglobulins, although myeloma is exceedingly unlikely at this age; reduced levels of IgG and IgA are non-specific findings in those with heavy proteinuria
• Antineutrophil cytoplasmic antibody (ANCA): patients with ANCA-positive vasculitides can occasionally present with nephrotic-range proteinuria, but this would be unusual
• FBC and clotting screen: a renal biopsy will be needed.

Radiological tests

• Chest radiograph: this may show pleural effusions and is mandatory in the elderly nephrotic patient because of the association of malignancy with membranous nephropathy.
• Renal ultrasonography: in most cases, renal size will be normal or increased, the latter caused by oedema or infiltration (e.g. amyloid, diabetes).

Renal biopsy

• In children, minimal change disease accounts for over 90% of nephrotic cases and renal biopsy is reserved for those with renal impairment, frequent relapses or atypical clinical course.
• In adults, the range of causes of the nephrotic syndrome is much wider and renal biopsy is almost always recommended.

In this case the renal biopsy appearance was compatible with minimal change disease, meaning that histological

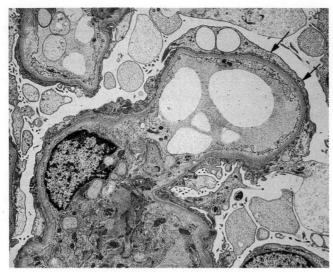

Fig. 3 Electron micrograph of glomerular changes in minimal change disease (×6200). Note the fusion of epithelial cell foot processes (arrowed).

appearances were essentially normal by light microscopy and immunofluorescence, and electron microscopy showed only fusion of the foot process of the epithelial cell (Fig. 3) [3].

Management

Symptomatic

- Salt-restricted diet; fluid restriction is usually unnecessary
- Loop diuretics—usually oral furosemide (frusemide) or bumetanide (may be better absorbed from oedematous gut mucosa); resistant cases may require intravenous administration and/or addition of metolazone
- Intravenous salt-poor albumin may be used in resistant patients
- Monitoring fluid balance: daily weight is the best measurement, being much more reliable than fluid balance charts
- If the nephrotic patient is immobile, prophylactic subcutaneous heparin is indicated.

Specific disease-modifying therapy

The vast majority of cases of minimal change diseases are primary, it can be associated with drugs (e.g. non-steroidal anti-inflammatory drugs [NSAIDs]), malignancy (e.g. Hodgkin's lymphoma, thymoma, mycosis fungoides) and bee stings.

High-dose oral corticosteroids (1 mg/kg per day) usually lead to prompt resolution of proteinuria in minimal change disease. There is evidence that subsequent relapses are less likely if the initial course of steroids is continued for at least 2 (possibly 3) months rather than tailed down immediately on remission.

If relapses occur, they are treated with steroids. If relapses become frequent, or if patients cannot be weaned from steroids because proteinuria recurs as the dose is reduced, then second line-therapy is given—usually maintenance cyclosporin or a course of cyclophosphamide.

To avoid delay in treatment, known relapsers can be taught to test their own urine using dipsticks and initiate steroids after 3 consecutive days of 3+ proteinuria.

Prognosis of minimal change disease

Minimal change disease does not cause chronic renal failure. Acute renal failure, probably associated with acute tubular necrosis, is recognized during severe nephrotic relapses and in elderly people. Relapses are less common in adults than children, and may be stimulated by viral upper respiratory tract infection. Their frequency diminishes with time and in young patients with primary minimal change disease there is usually complete remission by the end of the third decade [4]. The exceptions include those who are eventually proven to have focal segmental glomerulosclerosis (FSGS) (see Section 2.3, p. 73).

1 Cameron JS. The nephrotic syndrome. In: Davison AM, Cameron JS, Grünfeld J-P, Kerr DNS, Ritz E, Winearls CG (eds) *Oxford Textbook of Clinical Nephrology* (2nd edn). Oxford: Oxford University Press 1998: 461–492.

2 Trompeter RS, Lloyd BW, Hicks J, White RHR, Cameron JS. Long-term outcome for children with minimal change nephrotic syndrome. *Lancet* 1985; i: 368–370.

3 Broyer M, Meyrier A, Niaudet P, Habib R. Minimal changes and focal segmental glomerular sclerosis. In: Davison AM, Cameron JS, Grünfeld J-P, Kerr DNS, Ritz E, Winearls CG (eds) *Oxford Textbook of Clinical Nephrology* (2nd edn). Oxford: Oxford University Press, 1998: 493–536.

4 Nolasco F, Cameron JS, Heywood EF, Hicks J, Ogg C, Williams DG. Adult-onset minimal change nephrotic syndrome. A long-term follow-up. *Kidney Int* 1986; 29: 1215–1233.

1.4 Rheumatoid arthritis with swollen legs

Case history

A 60-year-old woman with a long history of rheumatoid arthritis is referred by her GP because of recent onset of oedema (1 month) and 3+ positive dipstick proteinuria on two occasions. The creatinine is 170 µmol/L and the albumin 25 g/dL.

Clinical approach

The likely diagnosis, as in Section 1.3 (pp. 7–10), is the nephrotic syndrome, which should be confirmed with measurement of 24-h urinary protein excretion or spot urine protein/creatinine ratio.

This woman has impaired renal function: is this stable or is it deteriorating? It may be that previous monitoring indicates that the problem is long standing and stable, but a diagnosis needs to be made rapidly if it isn't. If you are not sure about this then you should either arrange for the serum creatinine to be measured again, to ensure no acute deterioration, or see the patient promptly to arrange investigation.

> Renal failure is best avoided. One measurement of serum creatinine:
> • does not mean that renal function is stable
> • cannot tell you if renal function is deteriorating.
> If creatinine is rising rapidly the tempo of the investigation should be very fast.

> Renal biopsy is not a substitute for history and examination.

History of the presenting problem

Most of the issues discussed in Section 1.3 (pp. 7–10) are equally applicable here, but there should be particular emphasis on the following:

• Is there anything to suggest chronic renal disease? As mentioned above, a previous serum creatinine measurement would be invaluable. But have there been previous abnormalities on urinalysis? A history of hypertension might also suggest a long-standing renal problem.

• Drugs: what medications are being taken now? What medications have been taken in the past? Ask specifically about over-the-counter drugs—patients don't always count them as medicines. In a patient with rheumatoid arthritis, remember particularly that NSAIDs can cause minimal change nephrotic syndrome (also acute and chronic interstitial nephritis—but these don't cause the nephrotic syndrome), and penicillamine and gold can both cause membranous nephropathy. This patient had been taking regular diclofenac and had previously been treated with gold.

• Activity of arthritis: how bad and for how long? As a generalization, the longer and the more active the arthritis, the greater the chance of secondary amyloidosis.

• Any other symptoms? The nephrotic syndrome, in particular caused by membranous glomerulonephritis, can be a complication of malignancy in the older patient. Is there any evidence of this? Has the patient lost weight? Has bowel habit changed?

• Any other symptoms? The presence of worsened constitutional symptoms with joint pains, rashes or night sweats might indicate the development of a vasculitis.

Examination

A thorough examination is required, paying attention to those aspects discussed in Section 1.3 (pp. 8–9), but also looking carefully for evidence of:
• Activity of arthritis
• Manifestations to suggest vasculitis—rash
• Malignancy—cachexia, pallor, lymphadenopathy, hepatomegaly?

Approach to investigations and management

Investigations

Approach is as in Section 1.3 (pp. 8–9), but note particularly in this case:
• Is the creatinine changing? If it is rising then renal biopsy is needed without delay.
• Serum immunoglobulins, serum and urine electrophoresis: plasma cell dyscrasias are common in this age group.
• Renal ultrasonography: necessary before a biopsy. Are there two normal-size, unobstructed kidneys? If both kidneys are small (<9 cm in length), this indicates chronic disease and biopsy is much less likely to reveal a treatable diagnosis.
• Chest radiograph: any suggestion of malignancy?
• Have a low threshold for investigation of gastrointestinal symptoms, which might indicate malignancy.
• Check faecal occult bloods; investigate if positive.

In this case the biopsy showed membranous nephropathy (Fig. 4) and no evidence of amyloid. The more common associations/primary causes of membranous nephropathy are the following:
• Infectious: hepatitis B
• Multi-system disorders: SLE
• Neoplastic: carcinoma (lung, colon, stomach, breast, other)
• Medications/toxins: gold, mercury, D-penicillamine.

There were no clinical or laboratory features to suggest malignancy or SLE. Gold had been stopped several years before and so the time course of events did not suggest that this was the culprit. Her membranous nephropathy was presumed to be idiopathic.

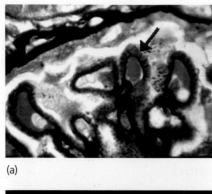

(a)

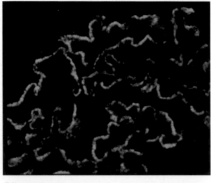

(b)

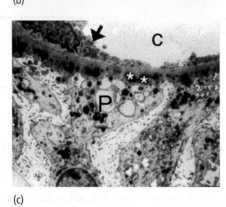

(c)

Fig. 4 Characteristics of membranous nephropathy: (a) silver-stained section. The basement membrane is widened, with spikes.
(b) Immunofluorescence for IgG. Part of the glomerulus is shown. There is granular fluorescence along the basement membrane.
(c) Electron micrograph of capillary loop. The basement membrane is seen adjacent to the capillary (C) lined by an endothelial cell (arrow). Within the basement membrane are electron-dense deposits (*). A podocyte (P) is also visible. (Courtesy of Dr D Davies, Oxford Radcliffe Hospitals.)

Management

Symptomatic

Management is as for Section 1.3 (pp. 9–10), but note the dangers of overdiuresis, particularly in older patients who can easily feel totally exhausted, develop postural hypotension with risk of falls and suffer acute deterioration in renal function. Hence:
• Aim for 0.5–1.0 kg weight loss per day (Fig. 5)
• Cut back on the diuretics if this is being exceeded
• Tell patients, particularly those given the powerful diuretic metolazone, to check their weight daily at home and omit/stop diuretics if they lose more than 1 kg/day.

> Furosemide (frusemide) is sequestered by albumin in the renal tubule, so high doses are often required in the nephrotic syndrome.

Disease-modifying therapy

The outcome of membranous nephropathy is difficult to predict:
• One-third go into remission
• One-third remain stable over time
• One-third progressively deteriorate, with rising serum creatinine.

In those who are deteriorating, treatment with cytotoxic agents can lead to improvement in some cases (Fig. 6).

Other management issues

ANGIOTENSIN-CONVERTING ENZYME INHIBITORS

Any patient with proteinuric renal disease and renal impairment will benefit from an ACE inhibitor to reduce proteinuria and the rate of progression of renal failure (Section 2.1.2, p. 50).

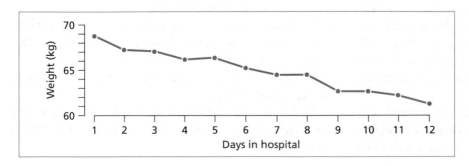

Fig. 5 Weight chart of a patient with nephrotic syndrome treated with intravenous diuretics (furosemide [frusemide] 160 mg once daily). Weight decreases at a satisfactory rate (8 kg over 12 days in hospital).

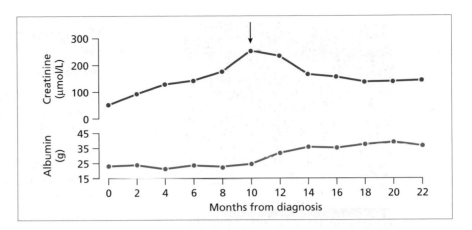

Fig. 6 Creatinine and albumin in a patient with membranous nephropathy. Renal function deteriorated progressively over 10 months from diagnosis and the patient was then treated with immunosuppression (intermittent chlorambucil and prednisolone for 6 months). This resulted in remission of the nephrotic syndrome and the creatinine returned to normal. The regimen used was based on that of Ponticelli *et al.* [1].

LIPIDS

Lipids are invariably deranged in the nephrotic syndrome, but the relationship to cardiovascular risk is not yet clear. There are animal data to suggest that lipid-lowering drugs may alter the course of progressive renal failure, but there are no reliable human data concerning this. Hydroxymethylglutaryl coenzyme A (HMG-CoA) reductase inhibitors reduce cholesterol effectively and should be considered if the nephrotic state persists.

RISK OF THROMBOSIS

There should be a high index of clinical suspicion when symptoms that could represent a thrombotic complication occur. Of particular note is renal vein thrombosis, which can present with the following:
- Flank/back pain
- Increasing proteinuria
- Haematuria: increased microscopic, sometimes macroscopic
- Rising creatinine.

If suspected, the diagnosis can be made by Doppler ultrasonography (requires considerable technical skill), computed tomography or renal arteriography (looking at the venous phase).

If any thrombosis does occur, then anticoagulation should continue for as long as the patient remains nephrotic.

ANTI-INFLAMMATORIES AND ANALGESICS

Remember that NSAIDs cause a fall in GFR. This does not cause clinical problems in those with normal renal function, but can do so when renal function is chronically impaired. If at all possible, this woman should avoid using them and take regular simple analgesics, e.g. paracetamol, for musculoskeletal pains.

Also note that opiates can accumulate in those with renal impairment, and regular doses of co-proxamol and similar agents could lead to nausea and drowsiness in this case.

 Glassock R, Cohen A, Adler S. Membranous nephropathy. In: *Brenner & Rector's The Kidney*, 5th edn (Brenner BM, Rector FC, eds.). Philadelphia: WB Saunders, 1996: 1452–1458.
1 Ponticelli C, Zucchelli P, Passerini P, Cagnoli L, Cesana B, Pozzi C *et al.* A randomized trial of methylprednisolone and chlorambucil in idiopathic membranous nephropathy. *N Engl J Med* 1989; 320: 8–13.

1.5 A blood test shows renal failure

Case history

A 38-year-old garage mechanic presented to his GP with a vague history of fatigue. He was pale and hypertensive (170/104 mmHg). Blood tests showed Na+ 134 mmol/L, K+ 4.8 mmol/L, urea 48 mmol/L, creatinine 1012 μmol/L, Hb 7.1 g/dL, mean cell volume (MCV) 89 fL, white blood cell count (WBC) 4.2 × 10⁹/L, platelets 254 × 10⁹/L. The patient was promptly referred to the local renal unit.

Clinical approach

Imaging of the renal tract is crucial. Urgent renal ultrasonography demonstrated small hyperechoic kidneys (8.2 and 7.8 cm) with no evidence of hydronephrosis. The subacute history, severely deranged biochemistry and small kidneys suggest chronic renal failure presenting at end stage, but note the following:
- There may be an element of acute-on-chronic renal failure
- If the ultrasonographic findings were incorrect, this might be reversible acute renal failure
- If renal failure is chronic, seeking the precise aetiology is often unrewarding.

End-stage renal failure in the unprepared patient can be completely overwhelming psychologically. The patient requires:

• An explanation of the situation
• A careful outline of the treatments involved, including details of when and how renal replacement therapy will be provided.

 Take an exhaustive approach before concluding that renal failure is chronic.

History of the presenting problem

How long has the patient had renal failure?

Renal failure does not produce dramatic symptoms. Ask specifically about:
• Energy: many patients with advanced renal failure simply notice that they are exhausted all the time
• Concentration: uraemia causes mental dulling
• Breathing: anaemia may cause breathlessness on exertion and fluid retention can cause pulmonary oedema
• Appetite, nausea or vomiting: uraemia causes anorexia and, when advanced, nausea and vomiting
• Nocturia: the normal kidneys elaborate concentrated urine at night; they cannot do this when they fail, leading to nocturia, a significant symptom in a young man or woman (prostatism being a much more common cause in older men)
• Itching: a symptom of uraemia.

Are there any clues from the past? Take a detailed history of any contact with medical services. Approach this from several angles:
• Have you ever had kidney disease or swelled up in the past?
• Has anyone ever taken your blood pressure before now?
• Have you ever had your urine tested?
• Have you ever had a medical for work or insurance purposes?
• Have you ever had a blood test or had blood taken?

Knowing that the creatinine was normal or abnormal 3 months ago could be crucial.

What is the cause of renal failure?

Explore all avenues that might suggest a diagnosis or aetiological factor. In particular:
• Recent illnesses such as diarrhoea or upper respiratory tract infection, which in retrospect may have heralded the start of the illness. These would favour an acute aetiology and should prompt re-evaluation of the clinical data.
• Multi-system disease? Any previous rashes, painful or swollen joints, eye pain, haemoptysis, numbness, weakness or tingling—these may point to a systemic inflammatory illness such as vasculitis (see Section 2.7, pp. 97–98).
• Urinary tract symptoms: childhood recurrent infections

or enuresis suggest reflux nephropathy (see Section 2.4, p. 85). Recurrent haematuria associated with upper respiratory tract infections could point to IgA nephropathy (see Section 2.3, p. 75). Has the patient had urinary stones?
• Drug history: this should include over-the-counter medications, illicit drugs, and traditional and herbal remedies because all of these have been known to cause renal failure.
• Family history of kidney disease or of deafness (see Section 2.8, pp. 102–104).

Examination

The overall clinical impression is valuable in differentiating acute from chronic renal failure.

 A patient who looks as sick or sicker than their blood results suggest most probably has acute renal failure.
The patient who appears rather well considering a grossly abnormal chemistry usually has chronic renal failure.

Take particular note of the following:
• Blood pressure
• Volume status: check lying and standing BP and height of the jugular venous pressure, listen to the lung bases and look for ankle and sacral oedema; if the patient has intravascular volume depletion, it is likely that renal function could be improved, although almost certainly not normalized, by rehydration
• Peripheral pulses and the presence of bruits
• Anything to suggest a multi-system disorder—skin lesions, arthritis, etc.
• Fundoscopy
• Urinary dipstick findings.

Approach to investigations and management

Investigations

In this case the history was in keeping with chronic renal failure presenting at end stage. The ultrasonographic examination was clear cut, showing small (right 8.2, left 7.8 cm in length), bright kidneys with no obvious cortex (Fig. 7).

Further pursuit of a specific diagnosis is likely to have a poor yield, make little difference in terms of subsequent management and potentially risk complications. In particular, a renal biopsy would not be useful. The investigations required are shown in Table 5.

 A renal biopsy is contraindicated in patients with small kidneys; it is technically difficult, has a high complication rate and the pathological findings are non-specific.

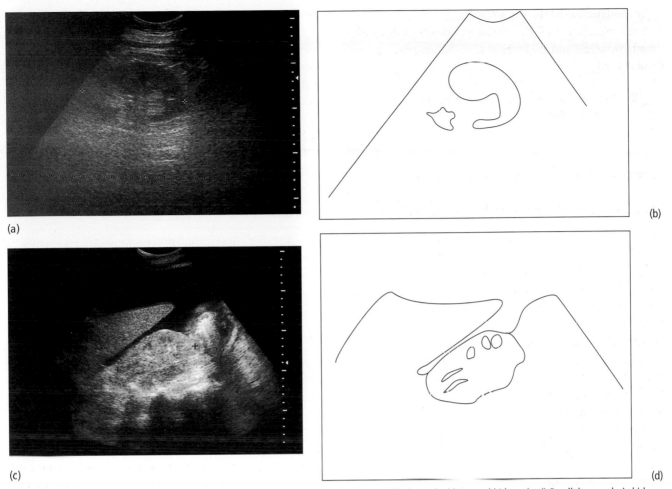

Fig. 7 Renal tract ultrasonography demonstrating the key features of chronically damaged kidneys. (a, b) Normal kidney. (c, d) Small, hyperechoic kidney without clear corticomedullary differentiation consistent with chronic renal failure.

Table 5 Investigations in the evaluation of chronic renal failure.

Investigation	Purpose
Full blood count and haematinics	Evaluation of contributory factors to anaemia
Calcium, phosphate, PTH	Assessing degree of secondary or tertiary hyperparathyroidism
Lipid profile	Cardiovascular disease is accelerated by CRF and is the main cause of death
Hepatitis B and C serology HIV testing (after counselling)	Positive patients will need specific haemodialysis arrangements. All patients who are HBsAg-negative should be vaccinated against hepatitis B
ECG and CXR	Evidence of LVH and/or IHD
24-h urine collection	The total volume may be useful in setting a level of fluid restriction

PTH, parathyroid hormone; CRF, chronic renal failure; LVH, left ventricular hypertrophy; IHD, ischaemic heart disease.

Table 6 Investigations to help exclude a possible acute aetiology.

Investigation	A normal result is likely to exclude the following diagnoses
Blood count and film	Haemolytic uraemic syndrome
CRP	Any inflammatory disease
Serum and urine electrophoresis	Myeloma
Anti-GBM	Anti-GBM disease
ANCA +/− ELISA for anti MPO or PR3	ANCA associated vasculitides
C3, C4, Auto antibody screen	Connective tissue diseases, SLE, MCGN, cryoglobulinaemia, infection-related glomerulonephritis

CRP, C reactive protein; ANCA, anti-neutrophil cytoplasmic antibodies; SLE, systemic lupus erythematosus; MCGN, mesoangiocapillary glomerulonephritis.

However, in some cases it is not certain whether renal failure is acute or chronic. It is then useful to carry out tests to rule out potentially reversible diagnoses (Table 6), and in some cases with relatively normal size kidneys a renal biopsy may be indicated.

If there is any doubt about ultrasonography, or it seems at odds with the clinical setting, ask an experienced radiologist to repeat the study or consider computed tomography, which is less operator dependent (Fig. 8).

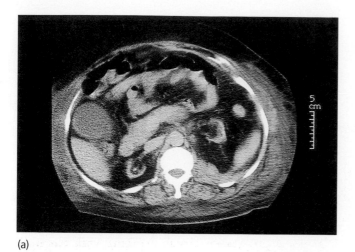

(a)

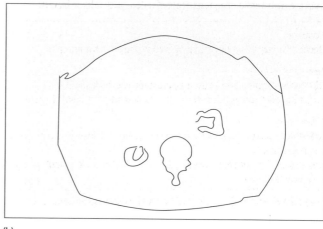

(b)

Fig. 8 Abdominal CT scan demonstrating small kidneys with little renal cortex, consistent with chronic renal failure.

Management

Information and support

Telling a patient that he or she has chronic renal failure and will need long-term renal replacement therapy can be devastating. The reaction is often similar to that seen in bereavement, with progression through shock, grief and denial before reaching acceptance. Accurate information and continued support are essential and best provided by a team which includes doctors, dietitians and specialist nurses.

Planning renal replacement therapy

Deciding what modality of dialysis to select depends on a combination of the clinical and social circumstances (see Section 2.2, pp. 61–72). Early entry on to the cadaveric transplant waiting list, or a living related transplant, is likely to be very desirable in this case.

Complications of chronic renal failure

Note the following:
• Cardiovascular morbidity and mortality are extremely high in patients on renal replacement therapy; all require a full cardiovascular risk assessment, followed by attempts aiming to deal with reversible factors such as smoking, hypertension and lipids
• Treatment of anaemia, usually with erythropoietin (see Section 2.1, p. 54)
• Treatment of hyperparathyroidism (see Section 2.1, p. 57).

 Stein A, Wild J. *Kidney Failure Explained*. London: Class Publishing, 1999. [This is an excellent guide to kidney failure written for patients. It gives a good idea of how information can be put across in a straightforward non-patronizing manner.]

1.6 A worrying ECG

Case history

A previously fit 74-year-old man presented to his GP after feeling unwell for 4 weeks. He had become anorexic with marked nausea and more recently vomiting. The patient was very breathless and there was a grossly enlarged bladder. The patient was referred to the surgical admissions unit where blood tests identified renal failure: Na^+ 134 mmol/L, K^+ 8.9 mmol/L, urea 72 mmol/L and creatinine 1208 µmol/L. The surgical house officer inserts a urinary catheter and asks for a medical opinion.

Clinical approach

 This patient has severe hyperkalaemia, a life-threatening complication of renal failure that requires urgent treatment. This should be instituted immediately, before extensive history taking or full examination.

The combination of renal failure with clinical evidence of urinary retention is usually the result of long-standing bladder outflow obstruction. This is most often caused by benign prostatic hypertrophy, although other possibilities should be considered (Table 7).

Bladder outflow obstruction with renal failure is a common clinical scenario, accounting for up to 30% of cases of acute renal failure in community-based studies. There is often a long history of urinary outflow symptoms and presentation is notoriously late.

Table 7 Differential diagnosis of renal failure with a large bladder.

Common
Obstructive nephropathy caused by benign prostatic hypertrophy

Less common
Obstructive nephropathy caused by prostatic carcinoma
Incidental acute urinary retention with another cause for renal failure

Uncommon
Obstructive nephropathy caused by a neurogenic bladder (e.g. Spinal cord compression*)
Obstructive nephropathy caused by other bladder outflow pathology e.g. urethral stricture

*see *Emergency medicine*, Section 1.23 and *Neurology*, Section 1.13.

Immediate action

> Treat first, ask questions afterwards.
> (Dr D Oliver)

Make a rapid initial assessment including overall clinical impression:
- Airway, breathing, circulation
- Which of four categories is the patient in: well, ill, very ill or nearly dead? If nearly dead, call for intensive care unit (ICU) help immediately—don't wait for cardiac arrest.

Sit the patient upright, give high-flow oxygen and ask nurses to prepare medical treatment measures for hyperkalaemia and pulmonary oedema. While this is being done, note the following:
- Can he talk?
- Is he exhausted?
- Kussmaul's breathing
- Cyanosis
- Respiratory rate
- Cold, shut-down peripheries
- Pulse rate

- Blood pressure
- Gallop rhythm
- Chest crackles or wheeze
- Pulse oximetry—oxygen saturation
- Arrange cardiac monitor
- Establish intravenous access
- Consider measuring arterial blood gases.

Hyperkalaemia

Diagnosis

The ECG is the best guide to the severity of hyperkalaemia. There are progressive changes starting with tented T waves, followed by diminished P waves with broadened QRS complexes, and finally a sine wave pattern before the onset of either asystole or ventricular fibrillation.

This patient's ECG showed a sine wave pattern (Fig. 9a) requiring immediate treatment.

Treatment

> If the ECG shows severe changes of hyperkalaemia:
> - diminished P waves
> - broadened QRS complexes
> - tented T waves
> give intravenous calcium immediately.

Treatments for hyperkalaemia are shown in Table 8.

SEVERE ECG CHANGES

Calcium counteracts the cardiotoxicity of hyperkalaemia by stabilizing the myocardium. It acts as soon as it gets to the heart, and its effect lasts for about 1 hour. It should be given intravenously in 10-mL aliquots, repeated as

Table 8 Treatment of hyperkalaemia.

Treatment	Dosage	Effect
Intravenous calcium	Calcium gluconate 10% in 10 mL aliquots iv slowly	Stabilizes myocardial cells and counteracts the cardiac toxicity of hyperkalaemia
Intravenous insulin and dextrose	10–20 units soluble insulin in 50 mL 50% dextrose infused over 20 min	Insulin induces cellular uptake of K^+ by activating Na/K-ATPase. Dextrose prevents hypoglycaemia
Nebulized β-adrenergic agents	Salbutamol 5 mg Neb.	Induces cellular uptake of K^+ by activating Na/K-ATPase
Oral or rectal ion exchange resins	Calcium Resonium 15 g oral tds	Removes K^+ from the body by binding in the GI tract. 1 g of resonium binds 1 mmol of K^+
Haemodialysis	2 h using dialysis fluid without K^+	Removes K^+ from the body by diffusion across semi-permeable membrane

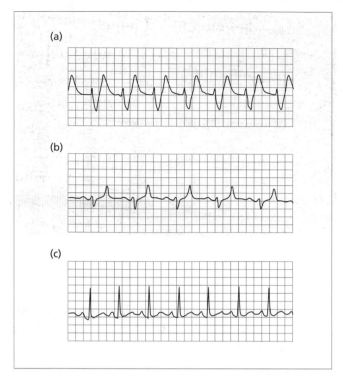

Fig. 9 ECG findings in hyperkalaemia: (a) initial ECG with [K+] 8.9 mmol/L showing a sine wave pattern: peaked T waves, broad QRS complex and absent P waves. (b) ECG after 40 mL 10% calcium gluconate: the P waves have returned and the complexes are starting to narrow. (c) Normal ECG after 2-h dialysis: serum [K+] 4.3 mmol/L.

Table 9 Indications for urgent dialysis.

Hyperkalaemia	Different patients respond differently to hyperkalaemia. If there are severe ECG changes then intervention is required
Pulmonary oedema	This is the commonest life-threatening manifestation of salt and water overload in acute renal failure. All patients should receive high-flow O_2 and be sat upright. Other holding measures while preparations for dialysis are made include intravenous nitrates, low-dose morphine and (in extreme circumstances) venesection
Uraemia	Severe uraemia (urea >50 mmol/L) is a relative indication. When associated with encephalopathy or pericarditis then urgent dialysis is required
Severe acidosis	This is usually a reflection of the severity of metabolic derangement and it is difficult to suggest a particular value for blood pH that demands intervention. A pH <7.2 should certainly prompt early intervention and dialysis

necessary, until the ECG improves significantly (Fig. 9b). Calcium does not affect the serum potassium concentration.

Then give insulin and dextrose and/or nebulized β agonist. These should lower the serum potassium by about 2 mmol/L for several hours.

LESS SEVERE ECG CHANGES

Give insulin and dextrose and/or nebulized β agonist. If acidosis is severe and there is no evidence of hypervolaemia or respiratory compromise, consider intravenous sodium bicarbonate.

Note that none of the treatments mentioned above actually removes potassium from the body. This can be accomplished by renal excretion, dialysis or to a limited degree by ion-exchange resins. In obstructive nephropathy relief of the obstruction will often lead to an immediate diuresis with potassium removal. When hyperkalaemia is severe, dialysis will often be necessary to remove potassium.

Pulmonary oedema

The spectrum ranges from mild breathlessness on exertion to respiratory failure leading to respiratory arrest. All patients should receive high-flow oxygen and be sat upright.

Those who are severely compromised with increasing respiratory rate, fatigue and hypoxia require transfer to the ICU and (probably) ventilation.

In others, intravenous nitrates may be sufficient until fluid can be removed by either:
• Diuresis—perhaps after the relief of obstruction in this case
• Dialysis with fluid removal by ultrafiltration.

Hyperkalaemia and fluid overload causing pulmonary oedema are the most common indications for urgent dialysis; others are given in Table 9.

History of the presenting problem

When appropriate, take a full history, concentrating on the following:
• Symptoms relating to renal failure: in this setting there is usually a non-specific prodrome with malaise, fatigue and sometimes nausea. As renal failure advances, these rapidly progress with the development of vomiting, confusion and eventually coma.
• Symptoms related to urinary outflow obstruction: chronic retention is usually painless in contrast to the restless agony of acute retention. Ask about frequency (most common and earliest symptom), urgency and difficulty with micturition (poor stream).
• Symptoms related to specific pathology: if obstruction is caused by pathology other than benign prostatic hypertrophy, then specific symptoms may be reported. Prostate or bladder malignancy may be indicated by loss of weight, haematuria or bone pain. Although almost certainly not the explanation in this man, kidney stones may be a problem in others.

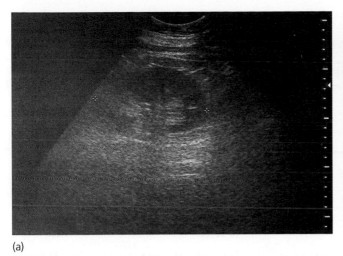
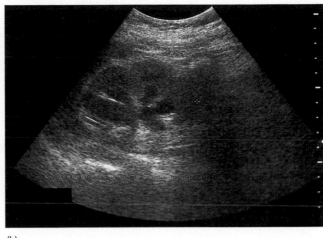

(a)   (b)

Fig. 10 Renal ultrasonography: (a) normal kidney; (b) hydronephrotic kidney with marked pelvicalyceal dilatation.

• Symptoms related to infection: urinary tract infection is present in at least 50% of patients presenting with renal failure caused by bladder outflow obstruction.

 If they are available, past biochemistry results indicate the chronicity of renal damage, and the level of recovery to expect. Check the notes. Check the path lab records. Ask the GP.

Examination

When the patient's condition permits, look for evidence of causal pathologies (see Table 7), especially:
• Lymphadenopathy, hepatomegaly—suggesting malignancy
• Rectal examination—benign prostatic hyperplasia or malignancy
• Neurological signs in the legs—this is unlikely to be bladder outflow obstruction resulting from spinal cord pathology, but it's a bad mistake to miss it.

Record the residual urine volume from catheterization and rate of urine output.

Approach to investigations and management

Investigations

Check the following:
• Full blood count
• Repeat electrolytes and renal function
• Liver function tests, calcium and phosphate
• Prostate specific antigen
• Chest radiograph
• Renal and bladder ultrasonography.

A large residual bladder volume in combination with bilateral hydronephrosis is diagnostic of obstructive nephropathy caused by a bladder outflow obstruction. This is most easily demonstrated by ultrasonography of the renal tract (Fig. 10).

Management

Involve the urology team at an early stage: the underlying problem is urological, but the medical complications demand immediate attention. Supportive measures and dialysis should be administered as required.

Fluid replacement

Relief of obstructive nephropathy is often followed by manifestation of renal tubular dysfunction. Diuresis can be profound and associated with bicarbonate, calcium, potassium and magnesium wasting. There is a risk of the patient becoming volume depleted, which could compromise recovering renal function. Note the following:
• Fluid status (postural hypotension, JVP and weight) and biochemistry should be checked frequently (usually daily)
• Care needs to be taken with the sodium content of intravenous fluid; alternating physiological (0.9%) saline and 5% dextrose is usually an appropriate choice
• Large quantities of potassium may need to be given (20–40 mmol/L); this requires close monitoring
• It is sometimes helpful to measure the urine biochemistry to determine the specific losses.

 Don't chase your own tail! Avoid driving a postobstructive diuresis with huge volumes of replacement fluid.

If the patient is polyuric, passing >3 L urine/day, give total fluid input equal to yesterday's measured output. This will achieve gentle negative balance, because insensible losses are not replaced. Monitor the response.

If renal function does not improve

The urethral catheter has drained the bladder, but there may be coincident ureteric obstruction. This is particularly common in prostate carcinoma, which can spread to encase the ureters. Repeat the ultrasonography to determine whether the hydronephrosis has been relieved. Consider computed tomography to look at the retroperitoneum.

The kidneys may have been chronically damaged by obstruction: sometimes long-term dialysis may be required.

There may be acute tubular necrosis (see Section 1.7) resulting from the combination of hypoxia, sepsis and poor perfusion. This is likely if the kidneys have good preservation of cortex.

Reconsider other aetiologies for the renal failure. How convincing was the evidence of obstruction and what was the residual urine volume? Look for other factors common in elderly people (e.g. evidence of myeloma). (See *Emergency medicine*, Section 1.15.)

Feest TG, Round A, Hamad S. Incidence of severe acute renal failure in adults: results of a community based study. *BMJ* 1993; 306: 481–483.

Firth JD. The clinical approach to the patient with acute renal failure. In: Davison AM, Cameron JS, Grünfeld J-P, Kerr DNS, Ritz E, Winearls CG (eds) *Oxford Textbook of Clinical Nephrology* (2nd edn). Oxford: Oxford University Press, 1998: 1557–1582.

Klahr S. The geriatric patient with obstructive uropathy. *Geriatr Nephrol Urol* 1999; 9: 101–107.

Sacks SH, Aparicio SAJR, Bevan A, Oliver DO, Will EJ, Davison AM. Late renal failure due to prostatic outflow obstruction: a preventable disease. *BMJ* 1989; 298: 156–159.

1.7 Postoperative acute renal failure

Case history

A 77-year-old man was admitted with a fracture of the neck of the right femur after a minor fall. He had experienced backache in the previous 2 years, which his general practitioner had treated as osteoarthritis. He also had mild angina. His operation was not unduly prolonged, but he required a 2-unit blood transfusion during surgery. Two days later, he was oliguric with a serum creatinine of 525 μmol/L, urea 28 mmol/L and potassium 6.3 mmol/L.

Clinical approach

The patient has acute or acute-on-chronic renal failure which can be distinguished on the basis of renal function at the time of admission.

Table 10 Conditions which may lead to acute tubular necrosis.

Pre-renal factors leading to renal hypoperfusion and ATN	Toxic ATN
Reduced circulating volume: blood loss; excess GI losses; burns	Rhabdomyolysis with urinary myoglobin
Low cardiac output states: toxic or ischaemic myocardial depression	Drugs: e.g. gentamicin; amphotericin
Systemic sepsis	Radio-contrast nephropathy
Drugs inducing renal perfusion shutdown: e.g. ACE inhibitors; NSAIDs	

ATN, acute tubular necrosis; ACE, angiotensin converting enzyme; NSAIDs, non-steroidal anti-inflammatory drugs.

The most common cause of acute renal failure is acute tubular necrosis (ATN) (see Section 2.4, pp. 80–81), which can be caused by a variety of stresses on the kidneys (Table 10). Several different factors often contribute [1].

Management depends on the identification and correction of causative factors (e.g. hypovolaemia, sepsis, nephrotoxic drugs or rhabdomyolysis), the assessment of the need for renal replacement therapy, and avoidance of unnecessary complications including hyperkalaemia and fluid overload.

History of the presenting problem

It is particularly important to establish whether the patient had pre-existing chronic renal failure:
- What was the serum creatinine on admission?
- Has serum creatinine ever been measured before?
- Has he ever had any kidney problems before?

Leads that need to be followed in this case include:
- Back pain: the previous history of this could indicate myeloma (see Section 1.14, pp. 40–43) or metastatic prostate cancer. These would be especially relevant if the femoral fracture was pathological.
- Drug history: the patient may have received non-steroidal anti-inflammatory drugs (NSAIDs) for back pain or postoperative analgesia. These can exacerbate intrarenal microcirculatory abnormalities during incipient acute renal failure (ARF), and also cause interstitial nephritis (not likely in this case, but see Section 2.4, pp. 80–81).
- Other underlying diseases: the patient had angina, must have arteriopathy and hence atherosclerotic renovascular disease is possible (see Section 2.5, pp. 86–87). Similarly, a previous history of diabetes, urinary tract symptoms (e.g. prostatic), etc. would be relevant.

Also, what happened before, during and after his operation? Assess the intra- and perioperative management. Look at the charts:
- What happened to his blood pressure?

• Was he given any potentially nephrotoxic drugs (e.g. NSAIDs antibiotics)?

Did anything else happen? Perioperative myocardial ischaemia or infarction could have occurred in this man. Has he had any chest pain? This could easily be missed in someone coming round from an anaesthetic and with pain from the wound.

Examination

Look in particular for the following:
• Circulation: is there hypotension? Is there intravascular volume depletion? Look for low JVP and postural hypotension (lying and sitting up, standing will not be possible). Is there volume overload? Look for raised JVP, crackles at the bases.
• Presence of sepsis: this is a major contributor to perioperative ARF; check wound, chest and urine.
• Bladder: does the patient have acute urinary retention?

Approach to investigations and management

Assess whether dialysis is urgently required (see Table 9).

In patients with renal failure, always make a rapid assessment of whether an immediate, life-saving intervention is required.

Investigations

The following investigations should be performed:
• Stick test of urine for blood and protein: it is most unlikely that this man has anything other than ATN, but the test is easy to do and there is a small chance that it could produce a surprise. Proteinuria trace/+ and haematuria trace/+ would not be surprising, but anything more should prompt urine microscopy and thought.
• Electrolytes and renal function: these should be monitored on at least a daily basis; indications for initiating planned dialysis include hyperkalaemia (e.g. potassium >6.5 mmol/L) or acidosis (pH <7.2).
• FBC, calcium and phosphate.
• Cultures: blood, wound swab, urine, sputum (if any).
• Check pulse oximetry.
• Chest radiograph: to identify pulmonary oedema or postoperative pneumonia.
• ECG: look for features of hyperkalaemia (see Section 1.6, pp. 16–19). Any evidence of a perioperative infarct?
• Urinary tract ultrasonography: in cases of ATN the kidneys are of normal size. A scan is necessary to exclude urinary tract obstruction, and small kidneys would signify pre-existing chronic renal disease.

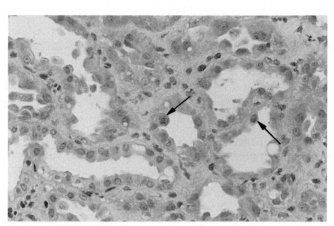

Fig. 11 Renal histological appearance of acute tubular necrosis. There are numerous necrotic tubular cells; mitotic figures (arrowed) indicate tubular cell regeneration (H&E, ×200).

Other specific investigations

Note the following:
• Serological tests to look for causes of nephritis are not appropriate in this case, but may be in other patients with indicative clinical picture.
• If the clinical picture fits with ATN, as it seems to do, then renal biopsy would not be performed. Biopsy would be indicated if there was genuine diagnostic doubt, when it might reveal the typical appearances of ATN (Fig. 11).
• Urine dipstick positive for blood but with no red cells visible on urine microscopy (Section 3.1) suggests rhabdomyolysis—confirmed by measurement of serum creatine kinase (test current and retrospective samples, looking for a very high value).

Management

Immediate management

Management consists of restoring the circulation, and identification and treatment of life-threatening complications (see Section 1.6, pp. 16–19) [2].

Sometimes renal function can be restored by vigorous haemodynamic management before severe tubular injury ensues. If urine output and renal function recover as soon as intravascular volume is restored, the diagnosis of prerenal uraemia is made. If they do not, then the diagnosis is ATN.

PRERENAL URAEMIA VS ATN

• The story: prerenal uraemia and ATN can be distinguished on the basis of urinary and plasma measurements. Table 11 is typical of that seen in many books.

Table 11 Urinary findings in ATN and prerenal uraemia: the story, not the truth.

	ATN	Prerenal uraemia
Urine sodium	>40 mmol/L	<20 mmol/L
Urine : plasma osmolality	<1.1 : 1	>1.5 : 1
Fractional sodium excretion (FeNa)*	>1%	<<1%
Urine : plasma urea	<7 : 1	>10 : 1
Urine volume	oligo-anuric or polyuria (recovery phase)	<1.5 L

*FeNa is the percentage of sodium that is filtered at the glomerulus (normally ~10 000 mmol/h) which actually appears in the urine (normal 6 mmol/h i.e. 0.06%).

• The truth: calculations based on measurement of urinary or plasma sodium concentration, urea concentration or osmolality do not separate patients into two groups, one with prerenal uraemia and one with ATN.
• The practice: few nephrologists routinely measure urinary electrolytes or osmolality in cases of acute renal failure. The distinction of prerenal uraemia from ATN is made retrospectively: patients have prerenal uraemia if they start to pass good volumes of urine after volume expansion; if they don't, they have ATN.

Continued management

After dealing with any emergency issues and starting fluid resuscitation (if needed), consider the following:
• Drug chart: are any nephrotoxins hidden away? Stop NSAIDs, ACE inhibitors and aminoglycosides unless there are really pressing indications.
• Urinary catheter: this will aid assessment of urine flow, indicating whether there is a response to treatment and assisting in the judgement of fluid requirements.
• Fluids: the amount of intravenous and oral fluids should be judged carefully. After immediate resuscitation to restore intravascular volume, give fluid volume equal to yesterday's fluid output plus allowance of 500–1000 mL for insensible losses. Assess volume status clinically at least twice a day and adjust fluid prescription in the light of this examination.

MEASURES TO INCREASE URINE FLOW

There is little evidence to suggest that loop diuretics and dopamine are effective in the treatment of ATN. They can increase urine flow, which may provide advantages for fluid and nutritional management. Some nephrologists use them and some don't. If they are to be used, then after restoring intravascular volume a reasonable scheme would be as follows:

1 Give frusemide (furosemide) 80 mg i.v. stat: no effect likely in someone whose renal function is significantly impaired
2 Start 'renal dose' (2.5–5 μg/kg per min) dopamine with high-dose loop diuretic (e.g. frusemide 250–500 mg, bumetanide 5–10 mg over 1–2 h)
3 Assess outcome after 2 h:
• if urine output not substantially altered, stop infusions
• if urine output has increased substantially, stop infusions and see what happens. If urine output then dwindles, restart dopamine and consider repeating frusemide up to a total dose of 1 g/day.

NUTRITION

Nutritional considerations are important in acute renal failure. Patients should receive oral or parenteral supplementation at an early stage [3].

RENAL REPLACEMENT THERAPY

When it becomes clear that renal replacement therapy will be required—usually because the urea and creatinine are rising inexorably day by day—there is no point in delaying until an emergency indication (see Table 9) develops. Indeed, it is dangerous to do so.

There is no good evidence on which to base recommendations, but it is generally agreed that early correction of uraemia may improve outcome by facilitating nutrition and helping to minimize extrarenal complications (e.g. pneumonia, gastrointestinal bleeding, sepsis and pressure area damage).

 As a rule of thumb, if the urea is rising from 30 towards 40 mmol/L, then arrangements should be made for dialysis; most nephrologists would agree that urea should not be allowed to rise above 50 mmol/L if at all possible.

Intermittent haemodialysis is the principal renal replacement therapy for patients with isolated ARF. Those with ARF as part of multi-organ failure are usually too haemodynamically unstable to tolerate this treatment and continuous replacement therapies, such as haemofiltration or haemodiafiltration, are used in the ICU [4]. Benefits include improved cardiovascular stability, optimal circulatory volume manipulation and the ability to create space for enhanced nutritional replacement.

Outcome in ATN

 A substantial number of old and frail patients who have ATN do not recover renal function.

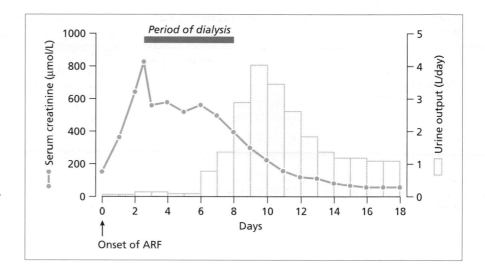

Fig. 12 Typical clinical course of acute tubular necrosis. After an initial oliguric phase, during which renal replacement therapy is sometimes necessary, renal functional recovery is often heralded by a period of polyuria.

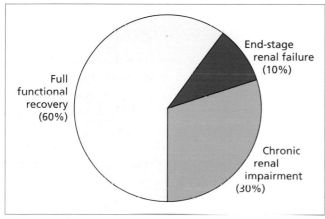

Fig. 13 Renal functional outcomes in patients who survive acute renal failure caused by acute tubular necrosis.

Firth JD. The clinical approach to the patient with acute renal failure. In: Davison AM, Cameron JS, Grünfeld J-P, Kerr DNS, Ritz E, Winearls CG (eds) *Oxford Textbook of Clinical Nephrology* (2nd edn). Oxford: Oxford University Press, 1998: 1557–1582.

1 Kleinknecht D. Epidemiology of acute renal failure in France today. In: *Renal Failure in the Intensive Therapy Unit* (Bihari D, Neild G, eds). Berlin: Springer-Verlag, 1990: 13–22.

2 Kalra PA. Acute renal failure. In: *Renal Disease: Prevention and treatment* (Raman GV, Golper TA, eds). London: Chapman & Hall, 1998: 293–324.

3 Feinstein EI, Massry SG. Nutritional therapy in acute renal failure. In: *Nutrition of the Kidney* (Mitch WE, Klahr, S eds). Boston: Little, Brown & Co, 1988: 80–103.

4 Bellomo R, Farmer M, Parkin G *et al.* Severe acute renal failure: a comparison of acute continuous haemodiafiltration and conventional dialytic therapy. *Nephron* 1995; 71: 59–64.

5 Bonomini V, Stefoni S, Vangelista A. Long-term patient and renal prognosis in acute renal failure. *Nephron* 1984; 36: 169–172.

The typical pattern of recovery in a patient with ATN is shown in Fig. 12.

Although most patients with ATN have potentially recoverable renal function (as tubular cell regeneration is likely), the overall prognosis for patients with ARF is poor: 55–60% of patients who require acute renal replacement therapy survive. This reflects the poor outcome of those who have ATN as a component of multi-organ failure: only 10–20% of those with failure of three or four organs will survive, compared with 90% of patients with ARF in isolation [5].

The renal functional outcome of patients with ATN is shown in Fig. 13. A substantial number of old and frail patients who have ATN do not recover renal function. An algorithm for the management of ARF is shown in Fig. 14.

1.8 Diabetes with impaired renal function

Case history

A man with type 2 (non-insulin-dependent) diabetes aged 58 is found to have hypertension (190/110 mmHg), proteinuria and creatinine 190 µmol/L.

Clinical approach

The most likely diagnosis is diabetic nephropathy, which accounts for 20–30% of all patients reaching end-stage renal failure.

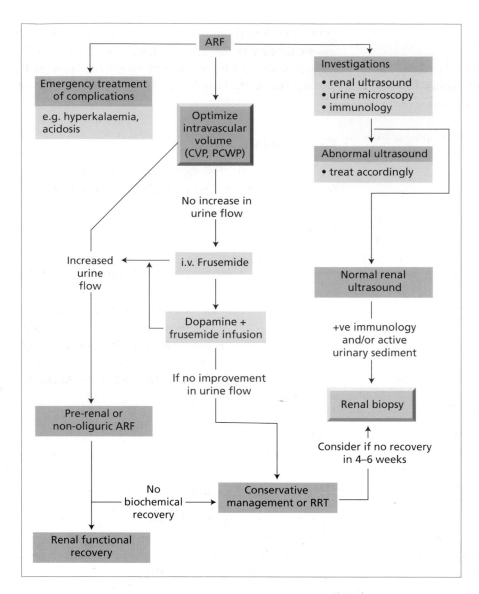

Fig. 14 Algorithm for clinical management of acute renal failure.

If the history, examination, and basic bedside and laboratory tests are all consistent with this diagnosis, it would be standard practice not to undertake further investigations, e.g. renal biopsy. The following are important questions:

- Could there be another (potentially treatable) cause?
- What (other) complications of diabetes does the patient have?
- How can the rate of progressive renal failure be minimized?

 Diabetic nephropathy is the most likely cause of proteinuria and renal impairment in a person with diabetes, but people with diabetes are not immune from other conditions.

History of the presenting problem

Key considerations

Diabetes and blood pressure

Some people with type 2 diabetes will have nephropathy at presentation, but usually this develops in those who are known to be diabetic. Hypertension and poor diabetic control are risk factors for the development of diabetic nephropathy. How long has there been hypertension? How is diabetes being monitored? How often is the patient actually testing blood sugar? What are the results?

 Glycosuria is not a measure of blood glucose in the presence of renal damage, when the renal threshold for glucose is lowered. This is generally appreciated in people with diabetes, but sometimes patients with other renal problems are noted to have glycosuria and the erroneous suggestion is made that they might have diabetes.

Renal impairment

Almost certainly creatinine will have been measured previously; if no result is immediately available, ask the patient if he or she has ever had a blood test, check with the labs and find out the results.

If renal impairment is long standing, it is unlikely to be reversible. If it is recent, or the duration is unknown, assume that it might be reversible.

Proteinuria

It is important to establish the duration of proteinuria. What do the records of the diabetic clinic and/or the GP show? Does the patient know? In diabetic nephropathy, the amount of proteinuria usually increases gradually and slowly over several years, typically starting with micro-albuminuria. Sudden onset of nephrotic range proteinuria would suggest a cause other than diabetic nephropathy.

Renovascular disease

Many people with diabetes have atheromatous vascular disease. Could renal vascular disease, which is potentially treatable, be responsible for hypertension and renal impairment in this case? Ask carefully for evidence of vascular disease and additional vascular risk factors:
- Angina
- Intermittent claudication
- Transient ischaemic attacks
- Previous vascular events—heart attacks, strokes
- Smoking history
- Family history of vascular disease.

Other diabetic complications

This is important in the general assessment of any person with diabetes, but note particularly that diabetic renal complications are rare in those who have diabetes but no retinopathy.
- Have they been treated for retinopathy?
- Are there symptoms of peripheral neuropathy?
- Are there symptoms of autonomic neuropathy?

Another renal diagnosis

This is unlikely in this case, but it is sensible to ask a few screening questions about other multi-system disorders and urinary obstruction. Ask specifically about rash, arthralgia, night sweats, urinary outflow symptoms and drugs.

Social history

It is more than likely that this man will be heading towards end-stage renal failure and dialysis within the next few years. You should certainly not tell him this at your first meeting, but you will need to know about his lifestyle, partner (if any) and home circumstances to be able to make informed recommendations about dialysis and other aspects of treatment in the future.

Examination

A complete and thorough examination is obviously required, but concentrate particularly on the following.

Cardiovascular

What is the blood pressure? Take again after 2 min and repeat until a stable reading is obtained. Record the average of the last two values. Is there postural change in blood pressure? This could be caused by intravascular volume depletion, vasodilatation or autonomic neuropathy. Where is the JVP? Is there oedema? Are the lung bases clear?

Is there evidence of vascular disease? Check the following:
- Foot pulses
- Carotid and femoral bruits
- Renal bruits.

Diabetic complications

Look specifically for the following:
- Foot ulcers
- Peripheral neuropathy
- Diabetic retinopathy (Fig. 15).

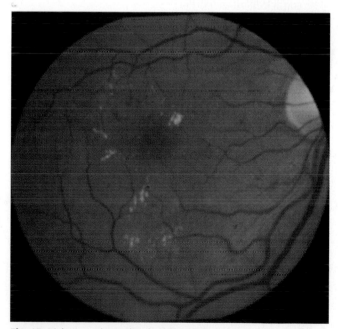

Fig. 15 Diabetic nephropathy: there are hard exudates and dot and blot haemorrhages near the fovea. (Courtesy of Dr P Frith, Oxford Radcliffe Hospitals.)

Blood pressure control is central to management of people with diabetes—especially those with nephropathy.

 Do you measure blood pressure in a reliable and reproducible way? The following are the key points:
- The patient should sit quietly for 5 min before BP measurement
- The arm should be supported at the level of the heart
- Bladder measurements: at least 75% of upper arm circumference and at least 50% of upper arm length
- Firm pressure will lower apparent diastolic BP; pressure from the stethoscope should be light
- BP tends to be raised by talking or being in a cold room; the room should be warm. Don't talk to the patient!
- BP should be taken at least twice—separated by 2 min. If there is more than a 5-mmHg difference, repeat the process until a stable reading is obtained.

- ANCA, anti-nuclear antibody, complement: simple screening tests for immunologically mediated renal damage.
- HbA_{1c} (glycated haemoglobin): a useful indicator or medium-term diabetic control.
- MSU: urinary infection is common in people with diabetes.
- ECG: evidence of previous myocardial infarction or left ventricular hypertrophy.
- Ultrasonography of the renal tract, looking for renal size: this is often normal, even with advanced chronic renal failure, in diabetes, but are both kidneys the same size? A disparity in length of more than 1.5 cm might suggest renovascular disease. Also look for presence of scars, evidence of obstruction and postmicturition residual.

 Older patients with unexplained renal impairment should always be screened for plasma cell dyscrasia.

Approach to investigations and management

Investigations

Is diabetic nephropathy an appropriate and sufficient diagnosis in this patient?

Bedside tests

Examine the urine—urinalysis and microscopy of the spun deposit. An active sediment suggests a diagnosis other than diabetic nephropathy.

Further investigations

- Biochemistry: is the creatinine changing? And how fast?
- Quantification of proteinuria: 24-h collection or test of spot urine sample for albumin excretion. This man clearly has renal impairment (creatinine 190 mmol/L) and almost certainly has diabetic nephropathy. If, as someone with diabetes, he had a normal serum creatinine, he would be categorized as having incipient diabetic nephropathy if the proteinuria were 0.2–0.5 g/24 h, urine albumin excretion rate (UAER) 30–300 mg/24 h, spot urine albumin 50–300 mg/l or albumin/creatinine ratio 10–25 mg/mmol. Values below these would be regarded as normal, and values above as indicating the presence of clinical nephropathy.
- Cholesterol and triglycerides: management of cardiovascular risk will be important. This patient will almost certainly benefit from cholesterol reduction.
- FBC.
- Protein and urine electrophoresis: plasma cell dyscrasias are a common cause of renal impairment in this age group.

Renal biopsy

In this case the history and clinical findings were entirely consistent with diabetic nephropathy:
- Eight years of diabetes mellitus
- + Proteinuria and creatinine 140 μmol/L recorded 1 year previously
- Known retinopathy
- No haemoglobin on urinalysis
- Both kidneys of equal and normal size on ultrasonography (right 10.8, left 11.1 cm in length)
- Electrophoresis: no monoclonal band in serum; urine shows generalized proteinuria.

It was considered that a renal biopsy was not necessary, given the very high likelihood of diabetic nephropathy and lack of pointers to other treatable diagnoses.

Renal angiography

There was a right femoral bruit. However, vascular disease is very common in patients with diabetic nephropathy (Figs 16 and 17). The following need to be taken into account:
- No renal asymmetry in this case
- Renal angiography carries significant risks
- It is unclear what the impact of angioplasty and/or stenting is on atheromatous renovascular disease in patients with diabetes.

A pragmatic approach, adopted in this case, was to treat with an ACE inhibitor and monitor renal function closely. This serves two functions:
- ACE inhibitors have been proved to slow progression of diabetic nephropathy

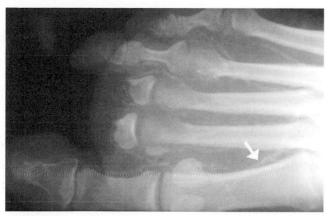

Fig. 16 Plain radiography of the foot in a patient with diabetic nephropathy. There is vascular calcification (arrow) and the second and third toes have been amputated.

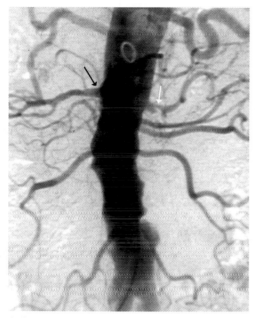

Fig. 17 Flush aortogram showing the renal arteries in a person with diabetes. The aorta is atheromatous. The left renal artery (white arrow) shows a 70% stenosis. The right renal artery is normal (black arrow). The left kidney was reduced in size (7.8 cm) and angioplasty was not attempted.

• Deterioration of renal function after ACE inhibition can be used as a functional indicator of significant renovascular disease. Check creatinine immediately before and 5–7 days after starting an ACE inhibitor. Frequently, creatinine will rise slightly, but a substantial rise (>20% from the basal value) is unusual and should result in the ACE inhibitor being stopped, and usually a renal angiogram being performed.

Management

Review drug therapies

The patient was being treated with metformin and bezafibrate at maximal doses. This is dangerous in renal impairment.

• Metformin carries an increased risk of lactic acidosis. Substitute glipizide, gliclazide or consider changing to insulin.

• Bezafibrate is renally excreted and accumulation increases the risk of myositis. As renal function is likely to continue to deteriorate, it is best to stop this drug. If lipid-lowering therapy is justified (likely), an HMG-CoA reductase inhibitor is safer.

In patients with renal impairment:
• Review all medications and their doses
• Tell patients to inform doctors and pharmacists giving them new medications of the fact that they have a kidney problem.

Blood pressure control

Control of hypertension in patients with diabetes reduces the risk of progression of renal impairment, and also mortality. In some patients, it can actually lead to stabilization of renal disease (Fig. 18). There is evidence that ACE inhibitors are particularly beneficial.

Note the following:

• Loop diuretics are often required to treat oedema.

• Aim for as low a BP as can be achieved and tolerated; three or more drugs are often required, and even then many patients fail to achieve a target of 135/85 mmHg (and some authorities would suggest that it was appropriate to aim even lower than this—perhaps 125/75 mmHg).

• Sodium restriction may be useful, and it can be helpful to measure 24-h sodium excretion to assess what the actual (rather than the perceived) salt intake is.

• Progression of diabetic nephropathy is more dependent on control of blood pressure than it is on the control of diabetes
• Always use an ACE inhibitor if this is tolerated
• Aim for as low a BP as can be achieved.

Cardiovascular risk factors

• If a smoker, encourage the patient to stop
• Encourage exercise
• An HMG-CoA reductase inhibitor will probably be justified.

Other aspects of managing chronic renal failure

• It is sensible to advise against NSAIDs
• Early prophylaxis against renal bone disease, e.g. with alfacalcidol 0.25 µg three times weekly
• Monitor renal function and, depending on rate of change, discuss and plan renal replacement therapy.

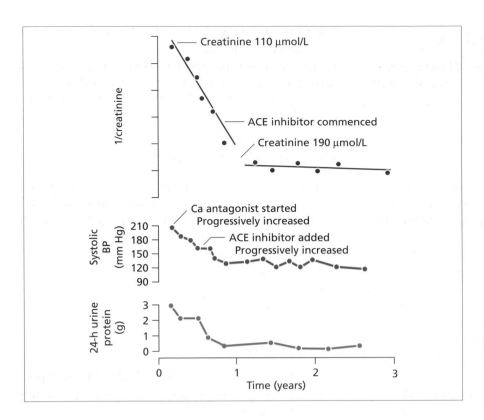

Fig. 18 Stabilization of course of CRF in a patient with diabetes. As blood pressure is controlled after introduction of an ACE inhibitor; GFR stabilizes and proteinuria is reduced. Such a good response cannot be anticipated in all patients.

Prognosis

Given the degree of proteinuria and the presence of significant renal impairment, this patient will almost certainly progress to end-stage renal failure. On dialysis, patients of this age who have diabetes have a mortality rate of at least 25% per annum.

Barnes DJ, Pinto JR, Viberti G. The patient with diabetes mellitus. In: Davison AM, Cameron JS, Grünfeld J-P, Kerr DNS, Ritz E, Winearls CG (eds) *Oxford Textbook of Clinical Nephrology* (2nd edn). Oxford: Oxford University Press, 1998: 723–776.

The sixth report of the Joint National Committee on prevention, detection, evaluation and treatment of high blood pressure. *Arch Intern Med* 1997; 157: 2413–2446.

UK Prospective Diabetes Study (UKPDS) Group. Intensive blood glucose control with sulphonylureas or insulin compared with conventional treatment and risk of complications in patients with type 2 diabetes (UKPDS 33). *Lancet* 1998; 352: 837–853.

UK Prospective Diabetes Study Group. Tight blood pressure control and risk of macrovascular and microvascular complications in type 2 diabetes: UKPDS 38. *BMJ* 1998; 317: 703–713.

Heart Outcomes Prevention Evaluation (HOPE) Study Investigators. Effects of ramipril on cardiovascular and microvascular outcomes in people with diabetes mellitus: results of the HOPE Study and micro-HOPE Sub-Study. *Lancet* 2000; 355: 253–259.

1.9 Renal impairment and a multi-system disease

Case history

A 26-year-old woman presents with several weeks of intermittent pleuritic chest pain and joint pain. The GP found proteinuria, a creatinine of 225 μmol/L and anaemia with fragments on the blood film. Renal referral was arranged.

Clinical approach

The first priority in a patient with pleuritic chest pain is to establish that the patient does not have pulmonary embolism.

Here the chest pain is not acute and the arthralgia, anaemia and impaired renal function all clearly suggest a multi-system disorder. The history and examination should elicit as much clinical information as possible. Simple tests such as urinalysis, plasma biochemistry and haematology often provide clues to the underlying pathology, its seriousness and the urgency of the situation.

Joint and chest pains in a young woman with renal impairment raise a strong clinical suspicion of systemic lupus erythematosus (SLE) (see Section 2.7.5, p. 95).

History of the presenting problem

Ask about the presenting symptoms and other possible manifestations of lupus. Renal disease is usually asymptomatic. Nephrotic patients may notice frothy urine and will (by definition) have oedema.

Joints

Ask which joints are affected, whether the distribution is symmetrical and whether it changes over time. Is there a diurnal pattern? Is there swelling, stiffness or discoloration? Is the pain eased or worsened by movement? These features are important in the differential diagnosis of arthritis (see *Rheumatology and clinical immunology*, Sections 1.10, 1.11, 1.18 and 1.19).

Other features of lupus

Ask for information regarding the manifestations shown in Fig. 19.
- Does the patient suffer from rashes or skin discoloration? Is his or her skin unusually photosensitive in the sun?
- Is there a history of thrombosis, spontaneous abortion or Raynaud's syndrome?

- Is there a history of neurological abnormalities, seizures or psychiatric disturbances?
- Have there been previous episodes of chest pain? Could these have been caused by pleurisy or pericarditis?
- Has the patient been taking any drugs? Some of these, e.g. hydralazine, can precipitate a lupus-like illness.

Consider pulmonary embolism

This is unlikely to be the diagnosis in this case, but it is always a very bad mistake to miss a serious (potentially fatal) and treatable disease. Although you anticipate the answer no to the following questions, ask about:
- Previous thromboembolism
- Leg/calf swelling
- Breathlessness
- Haemoptysis.

Examination

If the patient presented acutely with pleuritic chest pain, then the first priority would be to consider pulmonary embolism and look for:
- Signs of deep venous thrombosis in the legs
- Cardiorespiratory signs: raised JVP, palpable RV, loud

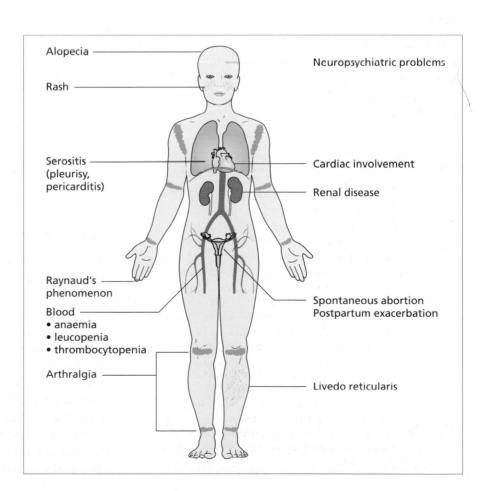

Fig. 19 Manifestations of systemic lupus erythematosus. This figure illustrates the widespread potential manifestations of this multi-system disease.

P2, RV gallop, pleural rub, pleural effusion (see *Cardiology*, Section 1.9 and *Respiratory medicine*, Section 1.5).

In this case look for the following:

• Skin: typically the facial butterfly rash and alopecia; also livedo reticularis.

• Joints: are these swollen or tender? Typically the musculoskeletal involvement in SLE consists of tendon contractures, myalgia and small joint arthropathy, which is symmetrical and usually non-deforming with no erosions.

• Fingers and toes: are there signs of ischaemia caused by severe Raynaud's phenomenon?

• Weight loss: SLE is a systemic disease.

• Cardiovascular: BP, signs of pleural or pericardial inflammation (rubs or effusions), cardiac murmurs, peripheral oedema.

• Neurological: are there any abnormalities?

Approach to investigations and management

 Joint pains, pleuritic chest pain and renal abnormalities should make you think of lupus.

The following are the requirements:

• To confirm or exclude rapidly (difficult!) the probable diagnosis of SLE

• To determine the nature of the renal involvement (see Section 2.7.5, pp. 95–97).

In this case, the symptoms alone would require some treatment, but the precise details of renal involvement will influence what form treatment takes.

Investigations

Urine

Around 10% of adults presenting with lupus have protein or blood in the urine, indicating renal involvement. Red cell casts confirm active glomerulonephritis. Proteinuria should be quantified (see Section 3.1, p. 106).

Biochemistry

Check renal function (to ensure no further acute deterioration in this case) and liver blood tests. Lupus can affect any organ, but liver involvement is unusual. Patients may have low serum albumin as a result of proteinuria and/or chronic disease.

Haematology

Check FBC, film, reticulocyte count, direct antiglobulin test (Coombs' test), clotting screen and haptoglobins.

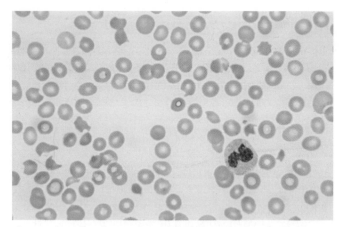

Fig. 20 Blood film of microangiopathic haemolytic anaemia. This blood film shows the typical features of a microangiopathic haemolytic anaemia with abnormally shaped red blood cells and red blood cell fragments. (Courtesy of Dr JA Amess, St Bartholomew's Hospital.)

Lupus often causes anaemia, which is usually normochromic and normocytic, but can be haemolytic. Haemolysis is suggested by a polychromasia, reticulocytosis, low haptoglobin levels and a raised unconjugated plasma bilirubin. A positive Coombs' test would suggest autoimmune haemolysis (see *Haematology*, Section 1.10). There may be abnormalities of clotting time as a result of antiphospholipid antibodies (see *Haematology*, Section 1.13).

In this case, the presence of fragmented red blood cells indicates a microangiopathic haemolytic anaemia (Fig. 20), the causes of which are:

• Pre-eclampsia or eclampsia

• Disseminated intravascular coagulation (DIC)

• Prosthetic heart valves, especially if leaking or infected

• Thrombotic, thrombocytopenic purpura (TTP)

• Haemolytic–uraemic syndrome (HUS)

• Accelerated phase hypertension

• Scleroderma

• SLE.

 Up to two-thirds of lupus patients have leucopenia, with the main deficit being lymphopenia. There may also be mild thromocytopenia. This contrasts with the primary systemic vasculitides, which usually cause high white cell and platelet counts.

Immunological tests and disease markers

The typical pattern of active lupus is a raised ESR with a low CRP, low levels of complement C3 and C4, antinuclear antibodies and antibodies to dsDNA. There may be other autoantibodies, especially antiphospholipid antibodies such as the lupus anticoagulants, which prolong the kaolin cephalin clotting time (KCCT) but paradoxically predispose to thrombosis (see *Haematology*, Section 2.4 and *Rheumatology and clinical immunology*, Section 3.2).

Renal ultrasonography

This is necessary as a prelude to renal biopsy. Are there two normal-size kidneys in the normal place? Reduced renal size suggests chronic damage.

Renal biopsy

Renal histology gives a guide to the renal prognosis and informs decisions about immunosuppressive management.

Management

 The only thing that is predictable about lupus is that it isn't.

Communication

Lupus is unpredictable; it can remit and relapse frequently. It can be a mere nuisance or it can be a devastating illness. This is worrying for patients; uncertainty is difficult for them, their family and friends, and also for their doctors. Many of the treatments used are of limited efficacy and have side effects. All these issues need to be frankly discussed with the patient at the beginning.

With women, discuss the interplay between pregnancy and lupus (and hypertension or renal impairment if present, see Section 1.2, pp. 5–7). Lupus can be exacerbated during pregnancy and for the first 2 months postpartum, and women with lupus have an increased incidence of abortion, perinatal death and pre-term birth.

Renal disease

Renal disease is treated with steroids and cytotoxic drugs, principally azathioprine and cyclophosphamide. The renal response to treatment depends on the histological appearances, e.g. lupus membranous nephropathy is usually not treated aggressively because it responds poorly. Studies from the US National Institutes of Health have shown benefit from steroid therapy in patients with severe diffuse proliferative lupus glomerulonephritis (Fig. 21). The benefit is increased if pulsed intravenous cyclophosphamide is added every 1–3 months. Plasma exchange offered no additional benefit.

Cyclophosphamide toxicity includes haemorrhagic cystitis, infection, bone marrow suppression, suppression of ovarian function and tumours. 2-Mercaptoethane sulphonate (mesna) helps protect against bladder toxicity.

 Drug toxicity should be discussed with the patient and, when practicable, storage of gametes should be considered before therapy is started.

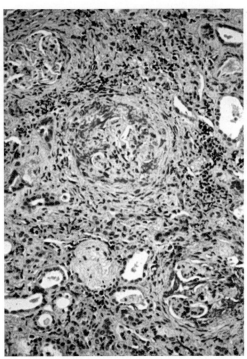

Fig. 21 Glomerulonephritis in systemic lupus erythematosus. This is a section of a renal biopsy showing a severe crescentic glomerulonephritis. The central glomerulus is full of inflammatory cells and shows a clear crescent caused by inflammatory cells in Bowman's space. (Courtesy of Dr JE Scoble, Guy's Hospital.)

Treatment of blood pressure is important. Dialysis and/or renal transplantation may be required if the kidneys fail completely.

 Austin HA, Klippel JH, Balow JE *et al.* Controlled trial of pulse methylprednisolone vs. two regimens of pulse cyclophosphamide in severe lupus nephritis. *N Engl J Med* 1986; 314: 614–619.
Cameron JS. Lupus nephritis. *J Am Soc Nephrol* 1999; 10: 413–424.
Lim CS, Chin HJ, Jung YC *et al.* Prognostic factors of diffuse proliferative lupus nephritis. *Clin Nephrol* 1999; 52: 139–147.

1.10 Renal impairment and fever

Case history

A 22-year-old man was admitted the previous day with fever and aching muscles. The creatinine on admission was 250 μmol/L. Urinalysis has shown proteinuria and haematuria. The question of a systemic vasculitis has been raised by the admitting team.

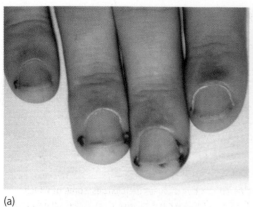
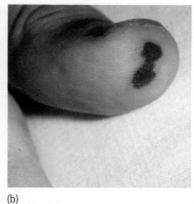

(a)　　　　　　　　　(b)　　　　　　　　**Fig. 22** Fingertip infarcts.

Clinical approach

The differential diagnosis of renal failure in this setting is very wide, but in a patient of this age it is usually possible to make a specific diagnosis rapidly. The following are important points:

• Creatinine 250 μmol/L indicates substantial impairment of GFR

• The patient may have a life-threatening condition but appear superficially well

• Take your own history (often something has been missed), examine the patient yourself and review all the available laboratory information

• Keep a completely open mind about the diagnosis—it could be systemic vasculitis, as suggested, but it could be sepsis.

 Even when glomerular filtration has stopped completely, serum creatinine will rise only by about 200 μmol/L per day.

History of the presenting problem

• 'How long have you been unwell?' Usually with systemic vasculitis, patients have been unwell for weeks or months. He says he became unwell 2 days ago.

• 'When were you last completely well?' The point is important enough to pursue; 22 year olds may be rather dismissive of more subtle symptoms.

• What did you first notice?

• Any recent travel?

• Recent symptoms of any kind?

Ask specifically about the following:

• Sore throat—poststreptococcal glomerulonephritis or IgA nephropathy

• Aching joints

• Skin rash

• Drugs (medicinal, recreational or alternative).

Examination

A thorough examination is required with the aim of:

• deciding how unwell the patient is (see Section 1.6, pp. 16–20)

• looking for signs to support a diagnosis of vasculitis

• looking for signs of sepsis.

Your overall impression is critical—how unwell is the patient? Is he well, ill, very ill or near death? If near death, call for ICU help immediately—don't wait for cardiac arrest.

Examination reveals:

• Temperature 39°C

• Pulse 110/min, regular

• Peripheries are strikingly warm

• Blood pressure 95/60 mmHg

• Infarcts around the finger tips (Fig. 22)

• Tender muscles.

These findings are very worrying indeed. They would be most unusual in a systemic vasculitis, as would the abrupt onset. The picture is more suggestive of a septicaemic illness, and the nail-fold infarcts raise the possibility of acute endocarditis. Aching and tender muscles are a common symptom in *Staphylococcus aureus* septicaemia.

Now repeat the history:

• Are you sure you haven't had any infections recently?

• No trouble with boils or spots?

• You haven't had an abscess anywhere?

• You haven't had bad toothache (or been to the dentist, although this presentation is not that of subacute infectious endocarditis, see *Cardiology*, Section 1.13)?

You repeat your cardiovascular examination—the pulse is too rapid to be sure of its character, but is there a decrescendo murmur?

 Patients who are ill often don't want to talk and get irritable when they are asked questions that they have been asked before. Don't be put off! You must repeat critical aspects of the history and examination. New information, or concern about a specific diagnosis, alters the threshold of suspicion for a particular feature.

Severe but acute aortic regurgitation may not be accompanied by an obvious diastolic murmur.

This man recalls that he had a spot on his elbow which burst a couple of days earlier. There is evidence of an infected olecranon bursa.

Approach to investigations and management

Your clinical diagnosis is acute endocarditis, probably staphylococcal. You need to confirm the diagnosis, institute appropriate supportive treatment and start empirical antibiotic treatment.

Keep the relatives informed—they need to know that this man could die.

Investigations

Can you confirm the diagnosis? Is existing information in support? Laboratory tests from the day before show a low platelet count, a neutrophil leucocytosis and a CRP of 300 mg/L.

Creatinine today is 400 μmol/L. Renal failure is likely to be contributed to by hypotension and the sepsis syndrome, but in addition it is likely that there is an active glomerulonephritis, as indicated by the proteinuria and haematuria. Renal complications in bacterial endocarditis include:
• Glomerulonephritis—similar to postinfectious glomerulonephritis histologically
• Acute interstitial nephritis
• Embolic events.
Arrange for the following:
• Blood cultures, and ask the bacteriology lab to check any previous cultures for growth. In this case, *Staphylococcus aureus* was grown from all the bottles
• Echocardiogram: this showed a bicuspid aortic valve, severe aortic regurgitation and a large vegetation
• Other blood tests: a test for ANCA was negative; complement levels (C3 and C4) were low (Table 12) as expected in acute endocarditis.

Management

In a life-threatening situation, it is often essential to start treatment before the diagnosis is confirmed. In addition

Table 12 Complement levels in glomerular disease.

Complement levels commonly low*	Complement levels usually normal
Postinfectious GN	IgA nephropathy / Henoch–Schönlein purpura
Lupus nephritis	Membranous nephropathy (unless associated with Hepatitis B or SLE)
Membranoproliferative GN	Anti GBM disease
Mixed essential cryoglobulinaemia	ANCA-associated vasculitides
Serum sickness	

*Also low in rare hereditary complement deficiencies, some of which predispose to SLE. In another rare circumstance there is a circulating IgG autoantibody that promotes complement breakdown, C3 nephritic factor, which is associated with membranoproliferative GN.
ANCA, antineutrophil cytoplasmic antibodies; GBM, glomerular basement membrane; GN, glomerulonephritis.

to antibiotics (see *Infectious diseases*, Sections 1.2 and 1.8), the following are appropriate here:
• Pulse oximetry, automated BP monitoring
• Give high-flow oxygen
• Urinary catheterization
• Move the patient to the ICU
• Central venous catheter
• Inotropic support.

After 48 h on the ICU, a decision was taken to operate and the patient's infected aortic valve was replaced (see Fig. 23). After surgery, recovery was uneventful, with renal function returning to normal.

Acute renal failure occurs in many severe illnesses. It is crucial to consider underlying diagnoses such as sepsis at an early stage. Approximately one-third of a series of 200 patients with bacterial endocarditis developed acute renal failure, which was more common in elderly people and those with a *Staph. aureus* infection [1].

Firth JD. The clinical approach to the patient with acute renal failure. In: Davison AM, Cameron JS, Grünfeld J-P, Kerr DNS, Ritz E, Winearls CG (eds) *Oxford Textbook of Clinical Nephrology* (2nd edn). Oxford: Oxford University Press, 1998: 1557–1582.
1 Conlon PJ, Jefferies K, Krigman HR, Corey GR, Sexton DJ, Abramson MA. Predictors of prognosis and risk of acute renal failure in bacterial endocarditis. *Clin Nephrol* 1998; 49: 96.

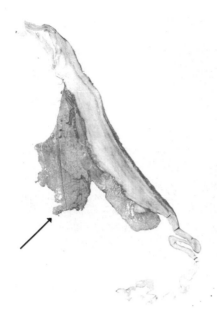

Fig. 23 Low-power view of section through the resected aortic valve leaflet showing adherent vegetation (arrow).

1.11 Atherosclerosis and renal failure

Case history

A 55-year-old man with peripheral vascular disease and hypertension started treatment with enalapril. Three weeks later, he went to his GP with a cough and shortness of breath. His creatinine was 450 µmol/L, whereas at the time of starting enalapril it had been 136 µmol/L.

Clinical approach

The history points to acute renal failure precipitated by an ACE inhibitor, in the context of renal artery stenosis caused by atherosclerotic renovascular disease (ARVD). Renal ultrasonography will be important to exclude obstruction and the finding of renal asymmetry would increase the likelihood of underlying renal artery stenosis.

 In addition to patients with ARVD, other groups are vulnerable to renal dysfunction with ACE inhibitors:
- Those with severe cardiac failure
- Those taking NSAIDs or loop diuretics
- Those who develop an intercurrent acute illness.

History of the presenting problem

The following are particularly important:
- Assess the severity of the peripheral vascular disease

- Establish whether the patient has a previous/current history of ischaemic heart disease or cerebrovascular disease
- Look for risk factors predisposing to vascular disease (e.g. diabetes, smoking)
- Drug history: NSAIDs and loop diuretics may be associated with renal functional deterioration when given in combination with ACE inhibitors.

Note also that patients with renal artery stenosis may suffer recurrent, sudden-onset, left ventricular failure—termed 'flash pulmonary oedema'.

Examination

How breathless is the patient? Does he need immediate removal of fluid, by haemofiltration if necessary? Probably not.

A full general examination is required, but note particularly:
- BP: 90% of patients with ARVD are hypertensive; many have primarily systolic hypertension associated with generalized arteriosclerosis
- Signs of overt cardiac failure, e.g. displaced apex beat, gallop rhythm, mitral incompetence
- Extrarenal vascular disease: the patient may have carotid or femoral bruits (in at least 60% of cases) and weak or absent distal leg pulses [1]
- Abdominal examination: auscultation may reveal epigastric or renal bruits (less common than femoral bruits); feel deliberately for a palpable aortic aneurysm
- Feet: acute renal failure can be precipitated by cholesterol atheroembolization, sometimes leading to mottling of the skin of the extremities (Fig. 24).

 Look for symptoms and signs of extrarenal macrovascular disease, which are usually present in those with atherosclerotic renovascular disease.

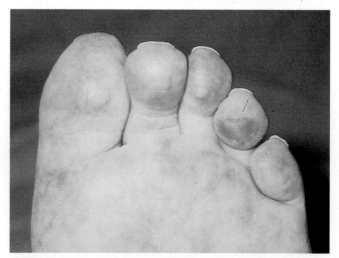

Fig. 24 Cholesterol embolization. Typical 'trash feet' and livedo reticularis appearance resulting from cutaneous ischaemia associated with distal embolization.

Approach to investigations and management

Stop the ACE inhibitor!

Investigations

Blood tests

These will include standard biochemistry (to ensure no further acute deterioration in renal function), blood count and, in any patient of this age presenting with renal failure, protein electrophoresis to rule out myeloma.

Urinary tract ultrasonography

The first-line imaging investigation for unexplained acute renal failure is ultrasonography of the urinary tract. In this case, the kidneys were 7.5 cm and 10.7 cm in length and not obstructed, further increasing the likelihood of significant renal artery stenosis.

Angiography and revascularization

Renal angiography was performed (see Sections 2.5 and 3.3, pp. 86 and 108) to confirm the diagnosis and assess whether revascularization was appropriate and technically possible. This showed a tight ostial stenosis (Figs 25 and 26) affecting his larger kidney, and he underwent angioplasty with a stent. The other artery had probably occluded previously.

Note that hypertension needs to be controlled, which may be dramatically easier after revascularization, and that interventions to reduce cardiovascular risk should be considered, e.g. aspirin, lipid-lowering agents.

OPTIONS FOR REVASCULARIZATION

These include the following:

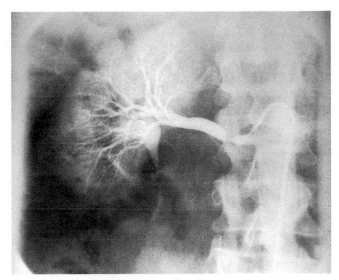

Fig. 25 Renal artery stenosis. Conventional intra-arterial angiography appearance.

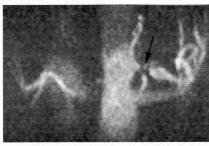

Fig. 26 Magnetic resonance angiography in the detection of renovascular disease. Note the proximal signal loss (arrowed), with poststenotic dilatation.

- Percutaneous transluminal balloon angioplasty (PCTA): low risk (complications of major bleeding or vascular occlusion in <1% of cases), but lesions close to the aortorenal junction (which account for 80–90% of all significant ARVD) have a high re-stenosis rate.
- PCTA with endovascular stent (Fig. 27): reduces rates of re-stenosis [2]. Complications are more frequent than with PCTA alone, and stents are relatively expensive.

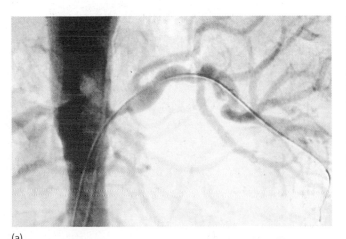

(a)

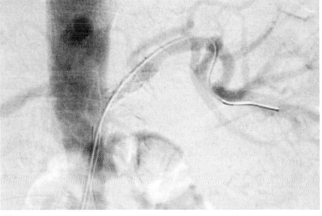

(b)

Fig. 27 Endovascular stenting in the treatment of renal artery stenosis. (a) Ostial renal artery stenosis. (b) After angioplasty, the stent has been placed in the proximal portion of the left renal artery, with the catheter passing distally into the intrarenal circulation. (Courtesy of Dr N Chalmers, Manchester Royal Infirmary.)

• Surgical revascularization: may be indicated in complicated disease, e.g. ARVD accompanying an aortic aneurysm, and where percutaneous techniques have failed.

Indications for renal revascularization in atherosclerotic renovascular disease are controversial, but it should be considered for patients with:
• Episodic flash pulmonary oedema
• Hypertension that is not controllable medically
• High-grade stenosis in artery supplying a single functioning kidney
• Stenoses and progressively deteriorating renal function.

WHY THE CONTROVERSY?

• There is no doubt that high-grade stenoses frequently progress to occlusion and that stenoses can be dilated or stented with high radiological success rates.
• There are few good-quality functional outcome data in ARVD: is hypertension improved? Does renal function improve or stabilize? How many patients really benefit?
• The risks: how many patients are made worse by fiddling?
• Where are the randomized controlled trials of optimal medical therapy with and without radiological intervention?

Conlon PJ, O'Riordan E, Kalra PA. New insights into the epidemiologic and clinical manifestations of atherosclerotic renovascular disease. *Am J Kid Dis* 2000; 35: 573–587.
Kalra PA. Atherosclerotic renovascular disease. In: *Horizons in Medicine*, No. 11 (Pusey C, ed.). London: Royal College of Physicians of London, 1999; 309–324.
Kalra PA, Kumwenda M, MacDowall P, Roland MO. ACE inhibitor usage and monitoring in general practice: the need for guidelines to prevent renal failure. *BMJ* 1999; 318: 234–237.
1 Choudhri AH, Cleland JG, Rowlands PC, Tran TL, McCarthy M, Al-Kutoubi MA. Unsuspected renal artery stenosis in peripheral vascular disease. *BMJ* 1990; 301: 1197–1198.
2 van de Ven PJG, Kaatee R, Beutler JJ *et al.* Arterial stenting and balloon angioplasty in ostial atherosclerotic renovascular disease: a randomised trial. *Lancet* 1999; 353: 282–286.

1.12 Renal failure and haemoptysis

Case history

A 66-year-old smoker experienced malaise, myalgia, arthralgia and increasing breathlessness for 5 weeks. One week before admission, he had haemoptysis and was given antibiotics by his GP. Over the following week, he became more short of breath. On return to the GP, a purpuric rash was noted and blood tests showed creatinine of 586 μmol/L and haemoglobin of 8.8 g/dL. Urgent renal referral was arranged.

Clinical approach

The clinical history suggests acute renal failure with pulmonary haemorrhage—a pulmonary–renal syndrome, the causes of which are shown in Table 13 [1]. The purpuric skin rash (Fig. 28) and prodromal syndrome suggest a systemic vasculitis. Other causes of haemoptysis should be considered, including bronchial carcinoma.

The patient sounds ill; diagnosis and treatment are needed urgently. If the history, examination and bedside tests support the presumptive diagnosis, immunosuppression should be started immediately, often before a histological diagnosis is made [2].

Although anaemia may suggest chronic rather than acute renal failure, this is unreliable. Pulmonary haemorrhage (as in this case), other bleeding or haemolysis can cause a low haemoglobin in acute renal failure.

Table 13 Causes of pulmonary renal syndrome.

Goodpasture's disease	Antiglomerular basement membrane disease
Primary systemic vasculitis	Wegener's granulomatosis Microscopic polyangiitis Churg–Strauss syndrome
Other systemic disorders	SLE Essential mixed cryoglobulinaemia Henoch–Schönlein purpura Behçet's syndrome (very rarely)

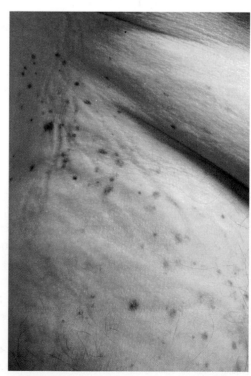

Fig. 28 Systemic vasculitis. Typical vasculitic rash in the axilla in microscopic polyangiitis.

History of the presenting problem

Look for clues to one of the diagnoses listed in Table 13.
• Antiglomerular basement membrane antibody disease can be triggered by inhaled hydrocarbons, and smoking predisposes to pulmonary haemorrhage
• Systemic vasculitis may occasionally occur in association with certain drugs (e.g. penicillamine, hydralazine or rifampicin), and with malignancy
• Wegener's granulomatosis would be suggested by a history of problems in the upper airways. Has there been chronic sinusitis, discharge or bleeding from the nose or ears?
• Asthma is a feature of the Churg–Strauss syndrome and Raynaud's disease may indicate cryoglobulins or other autoimmune rheumatic disorder, such as SLE.

Examination

How unwell is the patient? Is he well, ill, very ill or near death? If near death, call for ICU help immediately— don't wait for cardiac arrest. Assess need for immediate intervention, as described in Section 1.6 (pp. 16–17). Does he need ventilatory support, e.g. continuous positive airway pressure (CPAP) or ventilation? Does he need urgent dialysis?

A complete examination is obviously required, but think as you are doing it—is there any other evidence of vasculitis? In this patient, footdrop and loss of sensation in the distribution of the common peroneal nerve were found—a mononeuritis.

Approach to investigations and management

While beginning to investigate and manage:
• Monitor oxygenation (pulse oximeter) and circulation (regular vital signs) and be alert to the possibility of acute deterioration
• Give high-flow oxygen.

Investigations

The differential diagnoses of the pulmonary problem and renal failure must be narrowed rapidly. Aside from checking FBC, clotting, renal and liver function, blood cultures and blood gases, all of which are always appropriate in severe illness of unknown cause, the following are the key investigations:
• Urine dipstick and microscopy: the presence of proteinuria, haematuria and red cell casts confirmed an acute renal inflammatory process, i.e. nephritis
• Chest radiograph: look for appearances of pulmonary haemorrhage (Fig. 29), but remember that these cannot be distinguished with certainty from pulmonary oedema or infection

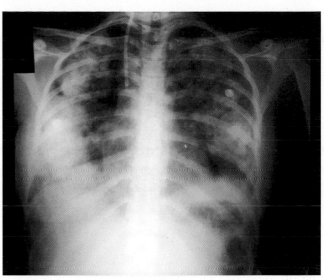

Fig. 29 Pulmonary–renal syndrome. Chest radiographic appearance of pulmonary haemorrhage.

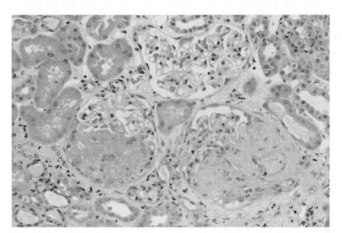

Fig. 30 Renal histological appearance in microscopic polyangiitis. Focal segmental proliferative glomerulonephritis (H&E, ×160).

• Renal ultrasonography: expecting to see normal-size unobstructed kidneys.

Given that the clinical and laboratory findings in this case were consistent with the diagnosis of a primary systemic vasculitis, immunosuppression was started while awaiting the results of testing for:
• Antineutrophil cytoplasmic antibody (ANCA)
• Antiglomerular basement membrane (anti-GBM) antibody.

This patient had a cytoplasmic ANCA (c-ANCA) titre of 1 : 512 (see below), consistent with primary systemic vasculitis (see Section 2.7.6, pp. 97–98).

Renal biopsy confirmed the diagnosis (Fig. 30) and was performed once the situation was stable, i.e. after dialysis has been given (if needed). Why do the biopsy at all? ANCA tests are not completely specific for systemic vasculitis, and biopsy can also give information about the likelihood of renal recovery, which may influence decisions concerning immunosuppression.

Pulmonary haemorrhage

Measurement of the KCO (carbon monoxide transfer factor) is useful in confirming and monitoring pulmonary haemorrhage. Intra-alveolar bleeding increases KCO, which can be very useful in distinguishing haemoptysis caused by pulmonary oedema from that resulting from pulmonary haemorrhage in patients with acute renal failure. In cases of severe pulmonary haemorrhage, there will be anaemia at diagnosis, and it is not unusual to see a daily fall in haemoglobin of 1–2 g/dL. Note, however, that KCO cannot be measured in those who are acutely ill (see *Respiratory medicine*, Section 3.6).

Immunosuppression

Initial immunosuppression in primary systemic vasculitis is with steroids and cyclophosphamide. In vasculitis (as opposed to anti-GBM disease), the role of plasma exchange is uncertain [3] (see Section 2.7.6, pp. 97–98).

Antineutrophil cytoplasmic antibodies

- These are directed against constituents of neutrophil cytoplasm: proteinase 3 (PR3) and myeloperoxidase (MPO)
- ANCA titres often reflect disease activity
- c-ANCA (cytoplasmic ANCA, anti-PR3): found in 90% of Wegener's granulomatosis patients and 40% of those with microscopic polyangiitis
- p-ANCA (perinuclear ANCA, anti-MPO): found in 60% of patients with microscopic polyangiitis and other connective tissue disorders
- Patients with classic polyarteritis nodosa are very rare, but usually ANCA negative.

1 Wilkowski MJ, Velosa JA, Holley KE *et al*. Risk factors in idiopathic renal vasculitis and glomerulonephritis. *Kidney Int* 1989; 36: 133–141.
2 Gaskin G, Pusey CD. Systemic vasculitis. In: Davison AM, Cameron JS, Grünfeld J-P, Kerr DNS, Ritz E, Winearls CG (eds) *Oxford Textbook of Clinical Nephrology* (2nd edn). Oxford: Oxford University Press, 1998: 877–902.
3 Pusey CD, Rees AJ, Evans DJ, Peters DK, Lockwood CM. A randomised control trial of plasma exchange in focal necrotizing glomerulonephritis without anti-GBM antibodies. *Kidney Int* 1991; 40: 757–763.

1.13 Renal colic

Case history

A 47-year-old man presented to the accident and emergency department with a 6-hour history of acute colicky loin pain, nausea, vomiting and haematuria.

Clinical approach

Organize appropriate analgesia, confirm the suspected diagnosis of a ureteric stone, and look for obstruction or infection. The possibility of an underlying stone-forming tendency needs to be considered.

History of the presenting problem

Symptoms from acute stone obstruction or passage of a stone are usually obvious. Sensory nerves from the ureter and renal pelvis enter the spinal cord at T11, T12, L1 and L2, and pain is referred to these dermatomes. The renal pelvis refers pain to the loin and back, the lower ureter to the testis or labium majus, and the lowest pelvic part of the ureter to the tip of the penis or perineum (Fig. 31).

Classic renal colic can scarcely be confused with any other condition, but when the pain does not radiate from the flank the differential diagnoses include the following:
- Musculoskeletal pain: usually not so severe; not typically associated with nausea or vomiting. Is the pain exacerbated by movement? Can the patient get into a comfortable position? Both of these features would strongly suggest a musculoskeletal cause.
- Biliary colic: typically felt in the right upper quadrant and epigastrium, and associated with nausea and vomiting. Is the pain brought on by fatty food? Has the urine gone dark and the stools pale? (See *Gastroenterology and hepatology*, Sections 1.6 and 1.3.)

Ask about the following:
- Haematuria (present in this case)
- Passage of grit, gravel or stones in the urine: which clearly would confirm the diagnosis
- Fevers, sweats, rigors: could there be infection, which with obstruction can be a deadly combination?

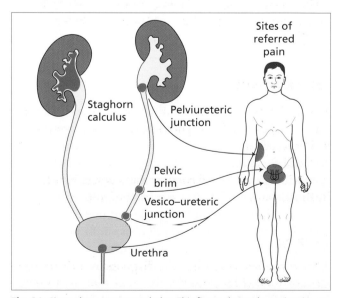

Fig. 31 Sites where stones can lodge. This figure shows the major sites at which urinary tract stones can lodge as they pass down the urinary system.

• Continued passing of urine: bladder stones can halt urine flow suddenly, with penile or perineal pain which is sometimes relieved by lying down.

Relevant past history

Have there been similar episodes previously? Ask carefully about predisposing factors:
• Family history
• Bowel disease
• Diarrhoea
• Use of antacids or vitamin D-containing compounds.

Examination

Look particularly for evidence of sepsis.

If the diagnosis is not certain, be sure to examine the following carefully:
• Spine and back: does movement exacerbate the pain? Is there local tenderness? Is the pain musculoskeletal?
• Upper abdomen: is there right upper quadrant or epigastric tenderness? Is this gall-bladder pain?
• Is the kidney tender?

Approach to investigations and management

The following are immediate priorities:
• Give adequate analgesia: NSAIDs, e.g. diclofenac, and/or opiates. Renal colic is terrible and yet some doctors are mean with the analgesia; there is no excuse for this at all.
• Maintain adequate hydration, if necessary with intravenous fluids.
• Exclude obstruction.
• Treat infection vigorously (if present).

 Stones can lodge in the ureter at the pelviureteric junction, at the pelvic brim or at the ureterovesical junction.

Investigations

• Dipstick test of urine: if there isn't at least a trace of haematuria, then the diagnosis of renal colic is in doubt
• Urine culture
• Renal function
• FBC: high white cell count would suggest infection
• Blood culture: if clinical suspicion of infection.

Imaging

This is needed to confirm the diagnosis of urinary stone disease, to demonstrate the site of any stone, to detect evidence (if any) of obstruction and to look for the presence of other stones.

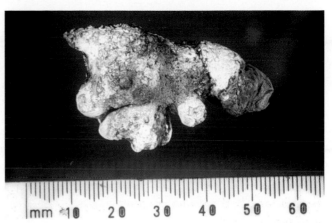

Fig. 32 A urinary tract stone. This is a huge staghorn calculus which was surgically removed from a patient. (Courtesy of Dr JE Scoble, Guy's Hospital.)

• Plain radiography: ask for a radiograph-KUB (kidneys, ureter, bladder): may show radio-opaque stones—calcium, cystine but not urate (Fig. 32).
• Ultrasonography: detects all stone types, and will demonstrate obstruction, but it is often difficult in the lower ureter
• IVU: will define the site of obstruction and the stone is usually visible as a filling defect.

Immediate management

Stones smaller than 6 mm in diameter usually pass spontaneously, but stones larger than 1 cm will not.

Obstruction with infection

This is an emergency requiring:
• Urgent (same-day) relief of obstruction, usually by anterograde percutaneous nephrostomy
• Broad-spectrum intravenous antibiotics pending culture results.

Obstruction without infection

This is usually diagnosed when ultrasonography shows dilatation of the pelvicalyceal system, but there are no clinical or laboratory features to suggest infection. Keep a watching brief if the patient's pain is controlled and the stone is likely to pass spontaneously (<6 mm diameter). If there is no progress over a few days, obstruction must be relieved—a range of techniques is available to urologists: extracorporeal shock wave lithotripsy, endoscopically, percutaneously or by conventional surgery.

Investigating reasons for stone formation

Reconsider the reason for stone formation only after the stone has been passed or removed. Go through the medical history again—has anything been missed?

Assess the patient's diet: do they eat large quantities of any of the following:

• Meat, fish and poultry: high in animal protein and purine
• Oxalate-containing food: rhubarb, spinach
• Salt and refined sugar: which together increase intestinal calcium absorption.

Note that, contrary to popular belief, high dietary calcium intake is not a strong risk factor for urinary stones, and the frequently given advice to cut out all dairy products can do more harm than good (see below).

Investigations

• Stone: analyse any stone passed to determine its constituents
• Spot urinalysis: pH, qualitative test for cystine (if radiolucent stone)
• Serum sodium, potassium, creatinine, urea, calcium, phosphate, albumin, urate, bicarbonate
• 24-h urine collection with acid preservative: volume, creatinine, calcium, sodium, potassium, phosphate, oxalate, citrate
• 24-h urine collection in plain container (no preservative): volume, creatinine, pH, protein, urate, cystine (qualitative test).

Look for an anatomical as well as a biochemical predisposition to stone formation—stone formation can occur because of urinary stasis, infection or around catheters. Ultrasonography is a good screening test for an anatomical abnormality.

> Hypercalciuria, usually idiopathic, is found in 65% of patients with urinary stones.
> Uric acid stones are almost always associated with abnormally low urine pH.

Further management

Further management depends on the type of stone and the reason for its formation (see Section 2.6.2, pp. 89–90), but the most important issue is that all patients who form urinary stones should be told to drink enough liquids to ensure a urine output of at least 2.5–3 L/day [1].

Also note the following:
• Do not advise patients to cut out all dairy products to correct hypercalciuria; a low dietary calcium intake causes an increase in intestinal absorption of oxalate and can thereby increase the risk of stone formation
• Advise patients with calcium-containing stones to avoid foods high in oxalate (not staple foodstuffs) and moderate animal protein intake if this is particularly high.

> Whatever the cause of the stones, increasing fluid intake always reduces the concentration of stone-forming substances in the urine and so reduces stone formation.

1 Borghi L, Meschi T, Schianchi T *et al*. Urine volume: stone risk factor and preventive measure. *Nephron* 1999; 81 (suppl 1): 31–37.

1.14 Backache and renal failure

Case history

A 60-year-old man presented with general malaise and lower backache. On examination, he was dehydrated and there was tenderness over his lumbar spine. Initial investigations showed plasma calcium of 3.2 mmol/L and creatinine of 275 μmol/L.

Clinical approach

The priority is to rehydrate the patient, control the hypercalcaemia and establish a diagnosis. The causes of hypercalcaemia are shown in Table 14. In this case myeloma seems the most likely diagnosis (Fig. 33), but other malignancies with lumbar metastases should also be considered.

History of the presenting problem

Symptoms related to hypercalcaemia

Hypercalcaemia can cause many symptoms, as listed in Table 15. Ask about these: they may give a clue as to how long ago problems began.

> Chronically high serum calcium levels cause neurological, gastrointestinal and renal symptoms (depressive moans, abdominal groans, renal stones).

Table 14 Causes of hypercalcaemia.

Common	Other
Primary hyperparathyroidism	Vitamin D excess
Malignancy–myeloma or metastases from solid tumour	Sarcoid or other granulomatous conditions
Chronic renal failure with complicating tertiary hyperparathyroidism	Immobilization
	Thyrotoxicosis
	Thiazide diuretics

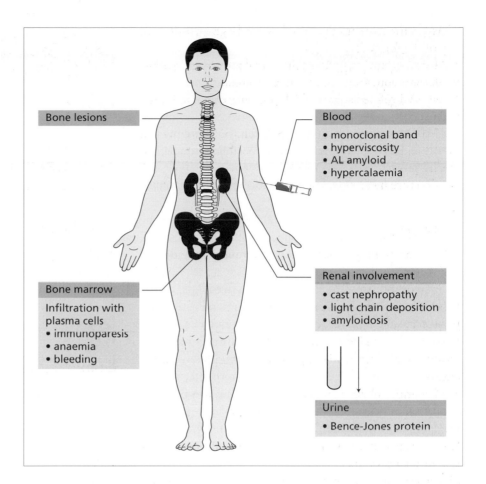

Fig. 33 Clinical features of myeloma. This figure illustrates the different ways in which myeloma can affect the patient.

Table 15 Symptoms and signs of hypercalcaemia.

Neurological	Drowsiness
	Lethargy
	Weakness
	Depression
	Coma
Gastrointestinal	Constipation
	Nausea
	Vomiting
	Anorexia
	Peptic ulceration
Renal	Nephrogenic diabetes insipidus and dehydration
	Stone formation
	Nephrocalcinosis
Cardiac	Shortening of the QT interval, sometimes with broad T waves and AV block
Others	Tissue calcification (may be detectable radiographically)
	Corneal calcification.

Symptoms related to causes of hypercalcaemia

Ask about:
• Weight loss—a general feature of malignancy
• Pointers to a primary tumour, e.g. haemoptysis, rectal bleeding, etc.

• Drug history: including over-the-counter medications and vitamin supplements, which many patients do not regard as drugs.

Examination

The following are important points:
• Assess hydration and circulatory volume carefully—is there a postural drop in blood pressure? What is the JVP? Are the lungs clear? Is there peripheral oedema?
• Is there any evidence of malignancy? Are any lymph nodes palpable? Check the breasts carefully. Feel for any abdominal mass or hepatomegaly. Do not forget rectal examination.

 Hypercalcaemia increases urinary sodium and water loss. This causes dehydration and a fall in GFR, which further reduces urinary calcium excretion.

Approach to investigations and management

You need to:
• treat the hypercalcaemia
• monitor renal function
• make a definitive diagnosis.

Treatment of hypercalcaemias

It is important to correct hypovolaemia and sodium depletion. This may require several litres of intravenous saline. When hypovolaemia has been corrected:
• Ensure that fluid input (oral or intravenous) is enough to encourage a urine output of 3 L/day, but monitor this closely and do not infuse large volumes of fluid into a patient who is anuric
• Consider giving a loop diuretic to increase urinary volume and calcium excretion.

If serum calcium remains very high (>3.0 mmol/L) or the patient continues to be symptomatic from hypercalcaemia, further therapy for hypercalcaemia might include the following:
• Bisphosphonates: the P-O-P bond of pyrophosphate is cleaved by a phosphatase during bone mineralization and in osteoclastic bone resorption. Bisphosphonates contain a P-C-P bond that is resistant to cleavage; they bind tightly to calcified bone matrix, impairing both mineralization and resorption. Use disodium pamidronate, up to a maximum of 90 mg by slow intravenous injection.
• Steroids: these are effective in hypercalcaemia caused by vitamin D intoxication, sarcoidosis and myeloma. They reduce calcium absorption in the gut, reduce the production of osteoclast-activating cytokines and can induce tumour lysis. They usually take 1–2 days to act.

Monitor renal function

If the renal impairment does not improve with rehydration and other measures to lower the serum calcium, it may require investigation in its own right:
• Check fluid input, urine output, daily weight
• Measure renal function and serum calcium daily.
  If renal function does not improve rapidly, then:
• Take a dipstick of urine and urine microscopy—proteinuria and haematuria would almost certainly indicate myeloma kidney, but could indicate another renal inflammatory lesion, e.g. malignancy-associated glomerulonephritis.
• Renal ultrasonography: what is renal size? Is there obstruction?

Establish the cause of the hypercalcaemia

The following would be the first tests to organize:
• Chest radiograph: are there bony secondaries? Is there lung cancer?
• FBC and film: is there anaemia? Are there rouleaux suggesting myeloma (Fig. 34)?
• Serum and urinary electrophoresis (monoclonal band): features of myeloma?
• Skeletal survey (lytic lesions): features of myeloma?

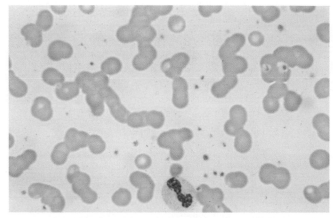

Fig. 34 Blood film of myeloma. This figure shows the peripheral blood film of a patient with myeloma. The red blood cells have formed stacks known as rouleaux. (Courtesy of Dr JA Amess, St Bartholomew's Hospital.)

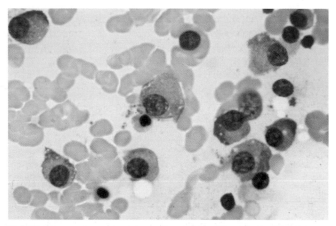

Fig. 35 Bone marrow appearances in myeloma. There are multiple nucleated plasma cells infiltrating the bone marrow. (Courtesy of Dr JA Amess, St Bartholomew's Hospital.)

• Examination of bone marrow (excess plasma cells—Fig. 35): features of myeloma?
  Any other leads should be followed:
• Parathyroid hormone (PTH) level will be suppressed by any cause of hypercalcaemia other than hyperparathyroidism. It will be high, or at the upper limit of the normal range (inappropriately so), in hypercalcaemia caused by hyperparathyroidism.
• In some patients with renal failure and myeloma, a renal biopsy is appropriate to determine how much irreversible damage has occurred.

 Alkaline phosphatase tends not to be elevated by myeloma deposits, but is increased in hyperparathyroidism and metastatic malignancy.

Management of myeloma

Note that the 1-year survival rate for patients with myeloma and end-stage renal disease is only 50%.

Hypercalcaemia and myeloma

Hypercalcaemia occurs in about 25% of patients with myeloma. Myeloma cells secrete osteoclast-mobilizing and -stimulating cytokines, and osteoclasts secrete interleukin 6 (IL-6) which is a growth factor for myeloma cells. Bone destruction is caused by osteoclasts related to collections of myeloma cells. Osteoblastic activity is reduced, so bone scans are usually negative in myeloma.

See *Emergency medicine*, Section 1.18; *Endocrinology*, Section 1.2; and *Haematology*, Sections 1.15 and 2.2.1.

Bushinsky DA, Monk RD. Electrolyte quintet: Calcium. *Lancet* 1998; 352: 306–311.

Clark AD, Shetty A, Soutar R. Renal failure and multiple myeloma: pathogenesis and treatment of renal failure and management of the underlying myeloma. *Blood Rev* 1999; 13: 79–80.

Winearls CG. Acute myeloma kidney. *Kidney Int* 1995; 48: 1347–1361.

1.15 Is dialysis appropriate?

Case history

A 78-year-old retired lecturer presented with acute shortness of breath. Three months previously metastatic carcinoma had been diagnosed. No primary site was identified and he was managed symptomatically with the involvement of community palliative care services. Investigations on this admission were consistent with pulmonary embolism.

On the fourth night, he was noted to be breathless, hypotensive, oliguric, confused and incoherent. Urgent blood tests showed K^+ of 7.2 mmol/L, urea of 62 mmol/L and creatinine of 422 μmol/L. Renal ultrasonography demonstrated normal-size unobstructed kidneys. The renal registrar was asked to review the patient with a view to offering dialysis.

Clinical approach

The impression is of a man who is dying and likely to do so within hours irrespective of any interventions. Making the positive diagnosis of dying can be helpful, allowing an appropriate change of emphasis. However, not all patients with incurable diseases who have renal failure should be refused dialysis. Decisions about whether to offer dialysis need to be made on an individual basis.

The first requirement is to assess the following:
- How ill is the patient?
- How much time is available to take a decision?

- Do you think that he would survive the insertion of access and a dialysis procedure?

It is bad medicine to perform futile and unpleasant procedures on patients during their final hours. Someone who is peripherally shut-down, breathing with difficulty and hypotensive will not last more than a few minutes on a dialysis machine.

The following are the next issues to consider:
- Does the patient really have metastatic carcinoma?
- How much better or worse would dialysis make the patient's immediate condition?
- Would additional time that might be provided by renal replacement therapy allow improvement in other factors?
- And, finally, can the patient be personally involved in any decisions?

Approach to investigations and management

Overall management strategy

- Make a careful assessment of current clinical state
- Assess the nature and prognosis of the terminal illness
- Consider the relationship between the terminal illness and the development of renal failure, and whether the renal failure is reversible
- Talk to other medical staff involved, the family and the patient (where possible)
- Always discuss matters with senior colleagues, but do not be forced into attempting treatment that you think is ill-judged, e.g. unkind or futile or both.

The patient who will die soon

If the patient is moribund (as in this case), decisions need to be made quickly. Trust your own judgement to make a decision based on your rapid bedside assessment and information from other involved medical staff, nursing staff and family members.

If the patient is dying, it is not kind or sensible even to speak to them about dialysis, but do not march out without saying anything to them. Hold their hand, and speak softly and kindly:
- The doctors looking after you asked me to see if I could help
- I will give them some advice
- I think that an injection (opiate) will help the breathing.
  If family are present, then speak to them:
- I am a doctor from the kidney unit …
- The doctors looking after your (relative) asked me to see him …
- His kidneys aren't working properly because he is dying …
- I am afraid that we cannot make him better …
- We must make sure that he's comfortable.

If they ask about dialysis, then reply:
• That's what the doctors on this ward wanted to know …
• It wouldn't help …
• He is not strong enough to stand a dialysis treatment …
• It would not do any good at all …
• In fact it might kill him sooner.

Never transfer intervention decisions to the family, and never leave them with the impression that:
• we could try a dialysis if you wanted us to …
• it wouldn't do any good …
• but we could give it a try.

Do not be afraid to take responsibility.

In this case, there was no doubt about the diagnosis of metastatic carcinoma. The patient's circulatory problems would not be improved by dialysis, which would be inappropriate and could even precipitate their demise. Symptomatic treatment was recommended and given, this being explained to the relatives.

When death is not imminent

If the patient were less ill than that described in this case, the situation would be different and there would be more time to take stock of the situation. Always discuss this sort of case with senior colleagues.

Nature and prognosis of the terminal illness

You need to decide the following:
• Are the key pieces of information correct?
• How certain is the diagnosis?
• What is the outlook in terms of symptoms, time and quality of life with and without dialysis?

Relationship between the terminal illness and the renal failure

Acute tubular necrosis, caused by hypotension and/or sepsis, is the most common cause of renal failure in patients with terminal illness. This is a potentially reversible condition, but only if the process causing it can be treated or removed. In the circumstances of a patient with a terminal disease, this often isn't possible, the development of ATN indicating that the underlying process is very advanced and not treatable.

Attempts to provide renal replacement therapy are usually inappropriate in this context: it is doubtful whether they prolong life, and it is certain that they adversely affect the quality of the life that remains.

Two specific scenarios should be noted:
• Obstruction: in patients with widespread malignancy, ureteric obstruction is not infrequent, and relief of this obstruction will often restore renal function to a level at which renal replacement therapy would not be required. Depending on other manifestations of the terminal condition, it might well be appropriate in this circumstance to give dialysis to a patient to get him or her into a state in which anterograde nephrostomy can be performed.
• In some situations, the renal failure can be directly related to the disease process, e.g. myeloma. The outlook is dependent on the specific disease and judgements must be made with this in mind.

Communication

Talking to the patient requires particular care and tact in this situation. It may be clear that the patient does want to talk about things, but this may not be obvious and they may prefer not to. You might begin with:
• I am a doctor from the kidney unit …
• Your kidneys aren't working well, and the doctors looking after you wanted to see if I could help …
• Are you keen to know exactly what's going on?
• Would you like me just to talk with your doctors and your (relative)?

If the patient does want to talk, and you think that it might be appropriate to attempt dialysis:
• The problem with the kidneys is this …
After a brief explanation of the details:
• We need to decide how best to deal with it …
• I need to review all the details and discuss things with my colleagues …
• There are a number of options, but I am wondering whether we should try to give you dialysis treatment….
After a further brief explanation:
• I am not sure whether this would help, but it might do …
• If we tried and it wasn't working then we would stop it, the same as any other treatment that wasn't working …
• The other options are that we use drugs to try to help the kidneys and the symptoms …
• What do you think about this?
Having got the patient's views:
• I will go and speak with my colleagues and come back to you (say when) about this.

Wherever possible, a consensus should be achieved, with the patient, relatives, doctors and nurses all aware of the decision and comfortable that it is appropriate. If there is genuine doubt, then dialysis should be offered, but it is bad medicine to try to put someone who is obviously perishing on to a dialysis machine. It is also fair to comment that doctors who do not work on renal units often have a much more optimistic view of what dialysis might achieve than those who do.

See *General clinical issues*, Section 3 and *Pain relief and palliative care*, Section 2.9.

 Higgs R. The diagnosis of dying. *J R Coll Physicians Lond* 1999; 33: 110–112.

1.16 Patient who refuses to be dialysed

Case history

A 70-year-old widower who is otherwise well has a creatinine of 700 μmol/L. He has never been keen on hospitals, and has told his GP that he does not want further investigations. The GP persuaded him to have renal ultrasonography, which showed small kidneys. Under pressure from his children, the GP has persuaded him to be seen at the local renal unit.

Clinical approach

First, ascertain that the facts are correct—that the creatinine is indeed 700 μmol/L and the kidneys are small—and the extent to which the patient is symptomatic. You should also assess the patient's general health and the presence of other conditions. If the patient has unsuspected disseminated carcinoma, then questioning his refusal of renal replacement therapy would be inappropriate.

But the problem here is an ethical one: can this man be allowed to refuse a treatment that would almost certainly prolong his life considerably? It may be tempting to divert from this with extensive history taking, examination and investigations, but it is more important to obtain the patient's trust and engage the central issue.

Why question the decision to refuse dialysis at all?

Renal replacement therapy is expensive and resources are limited, but it is well tolerated by most patients, especially in the absence of co-morbidity. Furthermore, older patients adapt well in psychological terms to renal replacement therapy, often better than younger patients.

Deliberately ignore other pressures. When human and financial resources are stretched, you may be more likely not to offer treatment, or to take a patient's refusal of treatment at face value.

Patients who do not follow medical advice are frequently put under a variety of pressures and made to feel very uncomfortable. Remember: in the first instance, doctors offer advice—the competent patient is at liberty to make his or her own decisions.

Approach to investigations and management

Talking with the patient

Remember the following:
• The patient is the person to decide what is right—your personal views, those of other professionals and of the relatives are of secondary importance
• Asserting your own view (or those of others) may be very unhelpful to a patient who is making a difficult decision.

However, while supporting the patient's right to decide, it is entirely appropriate to try to find out why they are making the decision to refuse further treatment. The duty of the doctor is to provide accurate and relevant information for the patient; they should not try to sell the patient treatment, but they should ensure that they have a realistic impression of what treatment could offer. The basis of the patient's decision may be entirely inappropriate, e.g. 'I am sure it wouldn't work at my age'. Try to understand the patient's viewpoint—this will put you in a better position to help.

Grounds for the decision

Look tactfully for the following:
• Competence: the patient may not be competent to absorb information and make a decision. This could be because of uraemia or other factors. If there is doubt about the patient's previous or current views concerning dialysis or the frame of mind in which he made his decision to refuse treatment, then it would be appropriate to offer firm advice that dialysis should be given. This is based on the grounds that, by so doing, you are keeping the patient's options open (by keeping him alive) and taking steps to put him in a position to make his own decision.
• Depression, e.g. following recent bereavement. Questions should be circumspect, but if you suspect that the patient's decision might be a manifestation of depression then you should arrange for urgent psychiatric review.
• Misconception of what dialysis involves: it is likely that the patient has no real understanding of this at all, in which case it is appropriate to spend time talking about the practicalities of haemodialysis and/or continuous ambulatory peritoneal dialysis (CAPD). Visiting the dialysis unit and meeting a dialysis patient of a similar age may be very helpful.
• Misplaced altruism: the patient may believe that if they accept treatment a younger person will not be treated [1].

Treatment on a trial basis

It may be helpful to point out that dialysis could be on a trial basis. Patients on dialysis can always withdraw from treatment—this is a common event whenever more elderly patients and patients with higher co-morbidity are taken on to dialysis programmes (e.g. in the USA).

Withdrawal from dialysis

In the USA from 1995 to 1997:
- Overall mortality rate on dialysis was 231 per 1000 patient-years
- Withdrawal from dialysis accounted for 41 of these deaths per 1000 patient-years
- Dying after withdrawal from dialysis was more common than death from septicaemia (25.2/1000 patient-years) or acute myocardial infarction (20.2/1000 patient-years).

Data from the US Renal Data System annual report 1999 [2].

In this case, the patient was undoubtedly competent to make his own decision and did not appear to be depressed, have misconceptions about dialysis or to be acting through misplaced altruism. He quietly but firmly persisted in his view that he did not wish to be dialysed.

Who else needs to be involved in the decision?

No one else need be involved in the decision. Ask the patient if he or she would like you to speak to the relatives, explaining that it is often helpful to do this. If possible, bring the involved parties (relatives, GP) round to support, or at least understand, the patient's point of view.

How should it be left?

Make it clear to the patient that he or she is entitled to a change of mind. When the time comes, the patient should be offered the same supportive care as if he or she were dying of any other condition. Involvement of the local hospice (if the patient wishes) would be entirely appropriate.

Elderly dialysis patients may cope better with the psychological stresses of dialysis than younger ones:
- This may be partly because older patients with co-morbidity or depression are selected against by being excluded from consideration for dialysis. However, at an age when death is not uncommon in the course of nature, dialysis can be considered to be a bonus.
- The young patient, by contrast, may see the need for dialysis in terms of limitation and loss.

See *General clinical issues*, Section 3 and *Pain relief and palliative care*, Sections 2.9 and 2.10.

1 Auer J. Psychological aspects of elderly renal patients. In: *Aspects of Renal Care 1* (Stevens E, Monkhouse P, eds). London: Baillière Tindall, 1986: 200–208.
2 http://www.usrds.org—The US Renal Data System (USRDS) is a national data system that collects, analyses, and distributes information about end-stage renal disease.

1.17 Renal failure and coma

Case history

A 34-year-old man was found unconscious 36 h after spending a night on a drinking binge with friends. On admission he was rousable but clinically dehydrated. He had tender, boggy swelling of the right leg below the knee, and the foot was discoloured but warm with palpable pulses. Biochemistry showed the following: urea 15 mmol/L, creatinine 430 μmol/L, potassium 7.2 mmol/L, phosphate 3.6 mmol/L, corrected calcium 1.85 mmol/L and venous bicarbonate 14 mmol/L. Dipstick urinalysis indicated haematuria, and the urine was dark brown.

Clinical approach

Acute renal failure in someone who is comatose can be the result of a number of insults, including hypovolaemia, drugs, sepsis and rhabdomyolysis; many aetiological factors often occur together.

The clinical presentation here strongly suggests that rhabdomyolysis is responsible for the renal failure [1], with the source of the muscle breakdown being compartments in the right leg, injured by ischaemic compression during coma. Drug overdose and excess alcohol are common contributors. The causes of rhabdomyolysis are shown in Table 16.

Supportive management, including dialysis, will be required. It is of the utmost urgency to relieve the compartment syndrome in the leg. Immediate surgery may be necessary to save the limb.

- Release of myoglobin and other constituents from ischaemic muscle can cause acute renal failure
- Serum potassium and phosphate rise rapidly
- Calcium is typically low
- Creatine kinase is massively elevated
- Serum creatinine may be disproportionately higher than urea.

Table 16 Causes of rhabdomyolysis.

Causes	Examples
Crush injury	Trauma or unconsciousness with compression
Ischaemic injury	Femoral artery thrombosis or embolism
Prolonged epileptic fits	
Drugs	HMG CoA reductase inhibitors
Overdose	Barbiturates, alcohol or heroin
Metabolic myopathies	McArdle's syndrome
Severe exercise	
Infections	Viral necrotizing myositis, coxsackie
Inflammatory myopathies	Polymyositis
Malignant hyperpyrexia	Certain anaesthetic agents
Hypothyroidism	

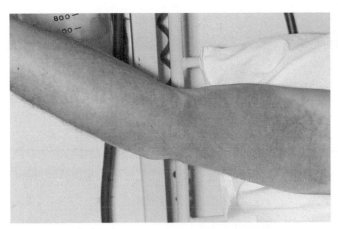

Fig. 36 Rhabdomyolysis. Swollen arm caused by muscle damage associated with trauma (in this case resulting from karate). If ischaemic compression is suspected, an urgent orthopaedic opinion should be sought as fasciotomy or débridement may be limb saving.

Examination

The first concerns in the assessment of anyone with coma are:
• Airway, breathing, circulation (ABC)
• Glasgow Coma Scale.

For details of how to deal with the comatose patient, see *Emergency medicine*, Section 1.26.

In a patient with suspected rhabdomyolysis, specifically examine the following:
• Muscle groups: look for evidence of swelling, tenderness and ischaemia (Fig. 36). Compartment syndrome refers to ischaemic compression, created by swelling within a muscle group that is constricted by fascial planes, resulting in necrosis of the muscle with or without compromise of the distal limb circulation.
• Limb circulation (particularly in the distal part of an affected limb): skin colour and temperature? Can you feel the pulses? Is sensation intact?

Look for evidence of any of the conditions listed in Table 16.

Underlying muscle disorders

Primary muscle disorders (e.g. metabolic myopathy or myositis) are rare, but they not infrequently present as rhabdomyolysis without a clear precipitant. Consider an underlying muscle problem, especially if the patient gives a history of intermittent or increasing muscular fatigue. Diagnosis is usually by muscle biopsy.

Approach to investigations and management

Investigations

Specific investigations will include the following:
• Urine dipstick and microscopy: the urine in rhab-domyolysis looks brown. The presence of myoglobin causes dipsticks to register strongly positive for blood on stick testing, but there are no red cells to be seen on microscopy.
• Serum creatine kinase: this will usually be extremely high, the absolute level giving some idea of the extent of muscle damage.
• Acid–base status: of relevance to treatment; myoglobin is more soluble in alkaline urine.
• Toxicology: in the comatose patient and/or where drug overdose is a possibility.
• Repeat electrolytes and renal function tests frequently (at least every 12 h): hyperkalaemia can develop rapidly in patients with rhabdomyolysis.
• Tests to look for evidence of any of the conditions listed in Table 16, as clinically indicated.

Management

The following are the immediate issues:
• Standard measures to manage the unconscious patient
• Correct intravascular volume depletion: give volume expander or 0.9% saline rapidly until the JVP is clearly visible
• Does the patient need immediate dialysis? (See Section 1.6, pp. 16–20)
• Insert urinary catheter to monitor hourly urine output
• Consider insertion of central venous pressure (CVP) line after volume depletion corrected.

Then proceed as follows:
• If volume expansion results in the patient passing good volumes of urine (>100 mL/h), maintain brisk diuresis (aiming for >100 mL/h). As myoglobin is more soluble in alkaline urine, it is common practice to induce an alkaline diuresis; this is often done using in rotation 500-mL bags of intravenous 0.9% saline, 1.26% sodium bicarbonate and 5% dextrose, each 500 mL given over 3 h [2].
• If volume expansion does not result in the patient becoming polyuric, do not continue to infuse large volumes of fluid—they will cause overload and pulmonary oedema—but arrange dialysis.
• Get surgical help quickly—compartment syndrome and ischaemic limbs may need fasciotomy, muscle débridement or amputation. These should be performed without delay.

1 Better OS. The crush syndrome revisited (1940–90). *Nephron* 1990; 55: 97–103.
2 Better OS, Stein JH. Early management of shock and prophylaxis of acute renal failure in traumatic rhabdomyolysis. *N Engl J Med* 1990; 322: 825–829.

2 Diseases and treatments

2.1 Major renal syndromes

2.1.1 ACUTE RENAL FAILURE

Abnormal renal function, identified by a high creatinine or oliguria (<30 mL/h), is frequent and caused by a wide range of processes. When it develops over hours or days, the term acute renal failure is used.

Aetiology/pathophysiology

Acute renal failure (ARF) can be caused by a problem anywhere from renal perfusion to the urethra. It is useful to classify by where the principal problem is—prerenal, renal or postrenal (Fig. 37).

Epidemiology

Transient renal dysfunction occurs in up to 5% of hospital admissions. Severe ARF in the UK (reversible increase in creatinine >500 μmol/L) has an incidence of about 140/million population per year.

Clinical presentation

Usually diagnosed on elevated plasma creatinine, or when oliguria develops in a patient whose urine output is being monitored reliably (e.g. catheterized). Sometimes the presentation will be a consequence of the renal failure (e.g. fluid overload or acidosis), but it usually relates to the underlying condition.

Immediate consideration must be given to whether dialysis (or another intervention) is required urgently. A circulatory assessment is essential.

In glomerulonephritis, there may be a nephritic presentation—meaning the combination of oliguria, hypertension, oedema and haematuria.

 Renal failure does not usually cause specific symptoms. Have a high index of suspicion in patients who are unwell for any reason and a low threshold for measuring serum creatinine.

Investigations

To assess severity/danger

The following are appropriate in all cases of ARF:

- Serum potassium and ECG (hyperkalaemia)
- Blood gases (PO_2 and pH) (oxgenation and acidosis)
- Chest radiograph (pulmonary oedema; other).

To determine the cause of the renal failure check the following:
- Examine the urine (blood, protein, casts)
- Renal ultrasonography (obstruction)
- Obtain results of any previous blood tests to prove that renal failure is acute
- Further investigations will be guided by the clinical setting (see Sections 1.6 [pp. 16–20], 1.7 [pp. 20–23], 1.9 [pp. 28–31], 1.10 [pp. 31–33], 1.11 [pp. 33–36], 1.12 [pp. 36–38], 1.14 [pp. 40–43] and 1.17 [pp. 46–47]). Many cases of ARF will merit renal biopsy to establish the diagnosis.

Note the following:
- Acute tubular necrosis: often the cause of ARF is prerenal failure/ATN. A renal biopsy will be performed only if there is doubt about the diagnosis.
- Obstructive uropathy will usually be diagnosed on ultrasonography. Be aware that occasionally rapid-onset obstructive uropathy, especially if the patient is volume depleted, may not result in hydronephrosis.
- Suspected renovascular disease/occlusion or renal vein thrombosis: renal angiography is the preferred investigation if renal failure might be the result of a renal artery occlusion/stenosis or renal vein thrombosis (usually in a patient with nephrosis).
- Blood tests will be helpful in certain settings, and in some circumstances will mean that a biopsy is not required, e.g. haemolytic–uraemic syndrome, disseminated intravascular coagulation, rhabdomyolysis.

Treatment

Urgent attention is given to maintaining oxygenation and the circulation. Determine whether immediate renal replacement is required.

 Indications for renal replacement therapy

- Hyperkalaemia (K$^+$ >6.5 mmol/L)—seriousness best evaluated by ECG (Fig. 38)
- Fluid overload not responsive to diuretic
- Acidosis
- Generally if urea >40 mmol/L (certainly if >50 mmol/L)

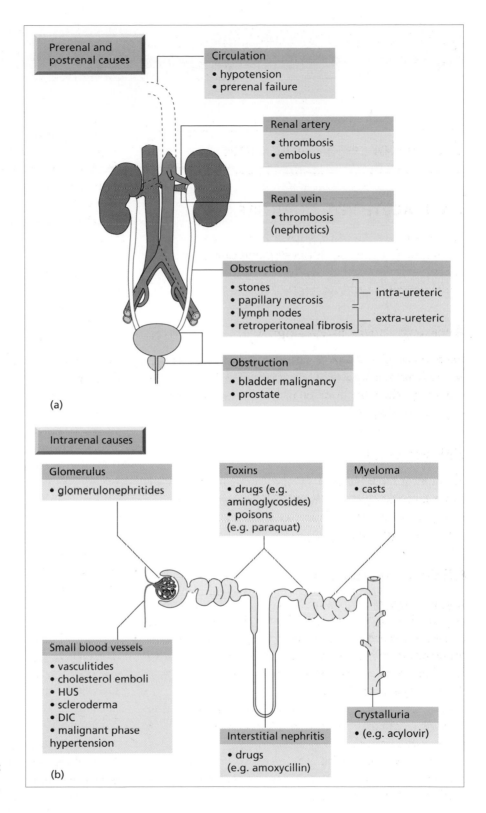

Fig. 37 Selected causes of acute renal failure:
(a) prerenal and postrenal; (b) intrarenal.

Acute renal failure is frequently a manifestation of very serious systemic illness. Sometimes—for instance, in the setting of disseminated malignancy—dialysis is technically feasible but may not be appropriate (see Section 1.15, pp. 43–44).

Supportive treatment

• Optimize the circulation (give fluid rapidly until JVP is seen easily, then stop and review the situation)
• Treat infection
• Avoid further renal insults (e.g. hypotension, nephrotoxic drugs)
• Maintain nutrition (enteral or parenteral if necessary)

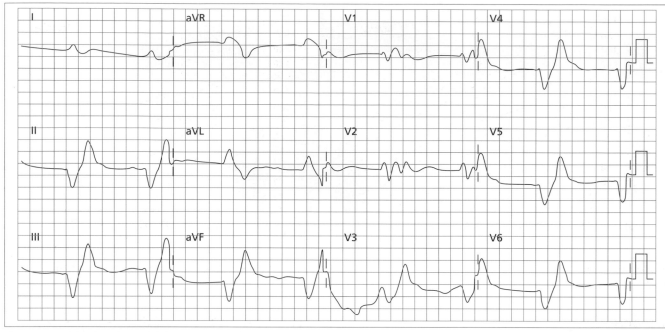

Fig. 38 ECG showing changes of severe hyperkalaemia. Widened QRS complexes slur into tall, tented T waves. There are no P waves. Cardiac arrest will occur soon if appropriate action is not taken immediately (see Section 1.6).

- Monitor fluid balance (input/output charts and daily weighing)
- Monitor renal function: biochemistry and urine output
- Renal replacement if necessary.

Treat underlying cause

See individual diagnoses in Sections 2.3–2.7 (pp. 72–102).

Prognosis

Mortality rate is about 40% in those requiring renal replacement therapy for ARF. It is much better when renal failure is not associated with other organ failure.

 Firth JD. The clinical approach to the patient with acute renal failure. In: Davison AM, Cameron JS, Grünfeld J-P, Kerr DNS, Ritz E, Winearls CG (eds) *Oxford Textbook of Clinical Nephrology* (2nd edn). Oxford: Oxford University Press, 1998: 1557–1582.

2.1.2 CHRONIC RENAL FAILURE

Chronic renal impairment is the irreversible loss of glomerular filtration rate (GFR). This is important for two main reasons:
- There may be direct consequences of impaired renal function
- Loss of GFR tends to be progressive, ultimately leading to end-stage renal failure.

Normal young adults have a much higher GFR (approximately 10-fold) than that needed for life, so substantial decrements in GFR often cause few (if any) symptoms.

 Don't dismiss a slightly elevated creatinine as a minor problem. In chronic renal impairment, lost nephrons cannot be recovered, and an elevated creatinine represents loss of about 50% of the GFR.

Aetiology/pathophysiology

Diverse primary processes result in loss of GFR (see Sections 2.3–2.7, pp. 72–102). The following are the most common causes in the UK:
- Glomerulonephritides (most common is IgA nephropathy)
- Diabetes mellitus
- Chronic pyelonephritis/reflux nephropathy
- Obstructive uropathy
- Autosomal dominant polycystic kidney disease
- Vascular disease/hypertension.

Loss of renal function tends to be progressive, probably from the following:
- Continuing loss of nephrons from the primary process (e.g. glomerulonephritis)
- Glomerular hypertension in remaining glomeruli—this increases GFR per nephron, but in the process leads to loss of further nephrons (hyperfiltration hypothesis).

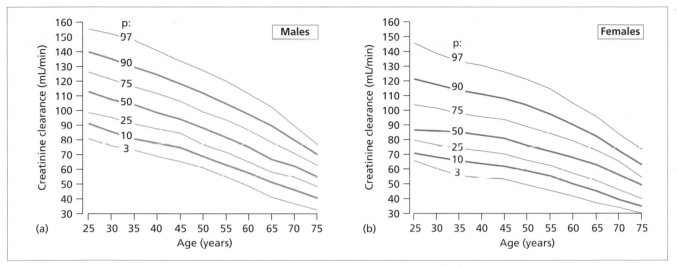

Fig. 39 Percentiles (p:) of creatinine clearances according to age and sex, calculated using the method of Cockcroft and Gault. (Redrawn from M.M.Elseviers *et al.* (1987) *Lancet,* i: 457.)

Epidemiology

Normal GFR in the population varies with age (Fig. 39), falling as patients get older. As muscle bulk (and thus creatinine production) also decreases, the normal creatinine remains the same. An elevated creatinine will be outside the normal range of GFR at any age, and usually represents loss of about 50% of GFR. In elderly people, a slightly elevated creatinine may represent a GFR of only 30 mL/min.

Investigation and interventions need to be considered in those who are outside the normal range for GFR and have risk factors for progression (hypertension, proteinuria), or when renal function is changing, even if the absolute value lies within the normal range. Prevention of progression is clearly most effective if started early, well before there are any symptoms attributable to renal failure.

Clinical presentation

- Most often with the incidental finding of a raised creatinine, abnormal urinalysis or hypertension
- Sometimes with symptoms related to underlying process (e.g. macroscopic haematuria, outflow obstruction)
- Symptoms/findings attributable to loss of renal function are often present in those with more severe renal impairment, but they are relatively non-specific, e.g. fatigue, anaemia, disturbed taste
- A significant number of patients will have previously unrecognized end-stage renal failure at presentation.

 Signs and symptoms pointing to chronic renal impairment rather than acute renal failure are commonly quoted but are very unreliable. Assume that any patient has acute (i.e. potentially reversible) renal failure until you can prove that it is chronic by finding a similar level of renal function months or years previously, or reduced renal size.

 Symptoms attributable to the loss of renal function occur late (GFR <25 mL/min). This has two implications:
- Check creatinine in high-risk populations (people with diabetes or hypertension, or those with dipstick protein or blood)
- In patients with moderately elevated creatinine (<300 μmol/L), symptoms need another explanation.

Investigations

To guide interventions

- Biochemistry (potassium, creatinine, calcium, phosphate)
- Haematological parameters.

Identify cause of renal impairment

If possible identify the cause of renal impairment, especially treatable conditions. All patients should have:
- Urinalysis and microscopy
- Renal ultrasonography.

Further tests are guided by these and the probable underlying cause in the particular patient. Choice of tests is also influenced by whether they could identify a treatable condition:
- Older patients should usually have serum and urine electrophoresis (Fig. 40)
- Patients with normal-size, unobstructed kidneys without scars should usually have a renal biopsy
- Those with small kidneys should not be biopsied: the hazards are substantial and no useful information can be obtained
- Monitoring renal function over time is important. Once creatinine is elevated (usually indicating loss of about 50% of normal GFR for age), serum creatinine alone gives a simple and reliable measure.

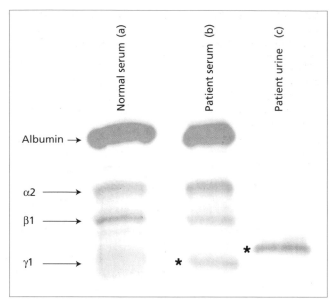

Fig. 40 Electrophoretic analysis of proteins in serum and urine. In the normal serum sample there is a broad gamma band containing IgA, IgG and IgM. In the sample from the patient there is a monoclonal band (*) which is an IgG κ paraprotein. In the urine there is a band which represents free κ light chain. (Courtesy of Dr S Marshall, Oxford Radcliffe Hospitals.)

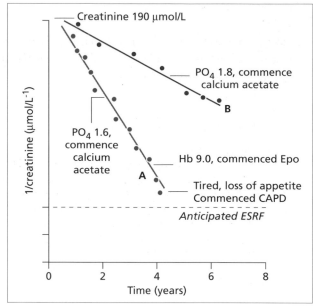

Fig. 41 Reciprocal creatinine plots against time for two patients with progressive chronic renal failure. Patient A had IgA nephropathy with protein excretion 3 g/24 h. Patient B had ADPKD.

 Once the creatinine is elevated, this gives a sensitive and straightforward indicator of changes in renal function, and it is not usually necessary to measure creatinine clearance. This avoids the inaccuracies and inconvenience of 24-h urine collections—many patients fail to collect all urine for precisely 24 h. If you try it for yourself, you will understand why!

 Often a reciprocal plot of creatinine against time is linear (Fig. 41), representing a constant rate of loss of GFR. This plot is useful in:
- Predicting when end-stage renal failure is likely to be reached
- Seeing whether a new value of creatinine is consistent with the expected trend. If a new value indicates a faster than expected deterioration, it may prompt a search for another cause (e.g. prostatic obstruction, urinary tract infection, NSAID).

Complications and treatment

Aims are to:
- prevent progression of CRF
- prevent secondary complications.

Where possible, the underlying cause of the renal damage should be treated or corrected (e.g. analgesic nephropathy, SLE, paraproteinaemia).

Progression of CRF

As stated previously, irrespective of cause, there is a tendency for CRF to progress.

 The amount of proteinuria correlates well with the risk of progression of CRF (Fig. 42).

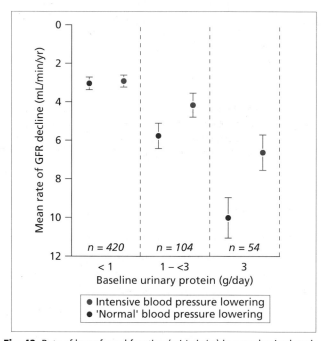

Fig. 42 Rate of loss of renal function (mL/min/yr) in a randomized study comparing a target mean arterial pressure of 107 mmHg with one of 92 mmHg. The patients were categorized according to the amount of proteinuria (g/24 h) [1].

Many interventions alter the course of CRF in animal models, including:
- Antihypertensives—especially ACE inhibitors which have a preferential action on the efferent arteriole, lowering glomerular pressure more than systemic blood pressure
- Protein restriction
- Lipid-lowering agents
- Antiplatelet agents

- Immunosuppression
- NSAIDs.

Antihypertensives are the only agents that have been proved to influence progression of CRF in convincing clinical trials in humans (see below).

Type 1 diabetes

In one study 409 patients were randomized to captopril or placebo. Other antihypertensives (but not calcium channel blockers or other ACE inhibitors) could be added. After 4 years of similar blood pressure control, the group given captopril had a slower rate of increase in plasma creatinine, and less likelihood of end-stage renal failure or death. In those with creatinine above 132 mmol/L, the rate of rise in the placebo group was 123 μmol/L/year vs 53 μmol/year in the captopril group. Importantly, there was benefit in normotensive patients [2].

Non-diabetic CRF

The Modification of Diet in Renal Disease was a 2 × 2 study of 840 patients, examining the effect of protein restriction; it also compared aggressive and standard BP control. Achieved mean arterial pressure in the groups was 91 and 96 mmHg (corresponding to 125/75 and 130/80, respectively). Benefit was greatest in those with more proteinuria (>3 g/day) and moderate renal impairment (see Fig. 42).

BP control is the only intervention that has been proved to slow progression of chronic renal impairment in humans. In patients with heavy proteinuria (>3 g/24 h) a BP of 125/75 is more beneficial than one of 130/80 (see Fig. 42).

Hypertension

A high proportion of patients with CRF (80% as end-stage renal failure approaches) will have hypertension. Treating hypertension slows progression, especially in those with proteinuria (see above), and is also presumed to reduce cardiovascular risk.

Treatment strategy

- Most are salt sensitive so it is appropriate to decrease salt intake.
- Many patients will require multiple antihypertensive drugs. First-choice antihypertensive is an ACE inhibitor (based on animal studies and studies of people with diabetes), excepting in those with renovascular disease.
- Loop diuretics (e.g. furosemide [frusemide]) are useful adjunctive agents, especially if there is evidence of sodium overload.
- In patients with proteinuria >3 g/24 h, target BP should be 125/75 mmHg.

Table 17 Foods and drinks high in potassium and some of their alternatives.

Foods and drinks high in potassium	Alternatives
Coffee	Tea
Fruit juice	Squashes
Beer, cider, sherry, wine	Spirits
Bananas, grapes, oranges	Apples, pears, satsumas
Chips, jacket potatoes	Rice, pasta
Baked beans, mushrooms, tomatoes	Carrots, cabbage, lettuce
Chocolate	Boiled sweets
Crisps and nuts	
Salt substitutes (e.g. Lo Salt)	

Hyperkalaemia

Hyperkalaemia will cause symptoms only at near lethal levels. Serum potassium should be monitored by blood tests (not symptoms!) and, acutely, ECG.

Treatment strategy

- Dietary restriction of intake (Table 17)
- Avoid potassium-sparing diuretics
- Consider changing from ACE inhibitor
- Correct acidosis
- In diabetes, improve diabetic control
- For emergency management, see Section 1.6.

Acidosis

Metabolic acidosis is usually a clinical problem only at or near end stage renal failure, and may contribute to feelings of malaise and breathlessness. Monitor venous bicarbonate.

Treatment strategy

- Avoid excessive protein intake
- Consider oral sodium bicarbonate, but sodium load may exacerbate hypertension
- Some patients will need dialysis.

Bone and mineral metabolism

As chronic renal failure progresses, phosphate excretion is insufficient and plasma phosphate rises, stimulating PTH secretion (Fig. 43). 1α-Hydroxylation of vitamin D (proximal tubule mitochondria) is impaired, which:
- de-represses PTH
- reduces calcium absorption and serum calcium, further stimulating PTH.

Consequences of elevated PTH

In normal individuals, this produces marked phosphaturia. In CRF, this does not occur, and phosphate rises as a result

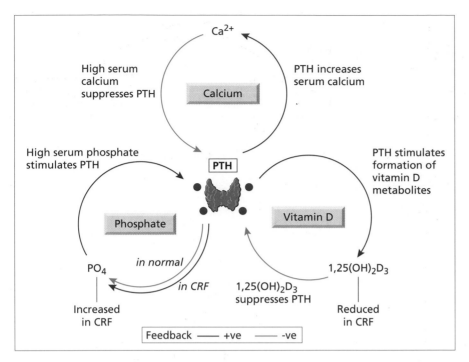

Fig. 43 The central role of the parathyroid gland in bone and mineral homeostasis, and the principal effects of chronic renal impairment.

of the increased bone turnover, further stimulating PTH. This results in the following:

- Bone loss with the risk of fractures
- Progressive parathyroid hyperplasia, and eventual autonomy
- Itching, calcinosis cutis
- Pyrophosphate arthropathy.

Treatment strategy

- Dietary restriction of phosphate.
- Phosphate binders, e.g. calcium acetate before food. Use of calcium is often limited by hypercalcaemia. Aluminium compounds are effective, but can cause toxicity as a result of accumulation. A new alternative, sevelamer hydrochloride, may reduce these problems but is expensive.
- Alfacacidol or calcitriol: corrects deficiency in activated vitamin D (Fig. 44). Use may be restricted by hypercalcaemia.

 Foods high in phosphorus

- Milk
- Eggs
- Cheese
- Yoghurt
- Cream

Anaemia

In renal disease, the renal cortical and outer medullary fibroblasts produce less erythropoietin for a given haematocrit. Consequently, the haemoglobin set point falls as GFR falls. The resulting anaemia is normochromic and normocytic (Fig. 45). Always consider other contributory factors, e.g. iron deficiency, ongoing inflammation.

Consequences include fatigue and left ventricular hypertrophy (LVH).

Treat with recombinant erythropoietin, which is usually not necessary until creatinine >400 μmol/L. Aim to maintain Hb >10.5 g/dL.

Cardiovascular risk, left ventricular hypertrophy

There is a high cardiovascular mortality in CRF—after correction for diabetes, age, sex and race, it is at least 10 times that for the general population once end-stage renal failure has been reached. Probable aetiological factors include hypertension, dyslipidaemia and elevated homocyst(e)ine.

Left ventricular hypertrophy is an independent risk factor for cardiovascular mortality and, as renal impairment progresses, the percentage of patients with LVH rises to 45% when GFR is <25 mL/min. Major factors are hypertension and anaemia.

Treatment strategy

- Attention to other cardiovascular risk factors (smoking and exercise)
- Meticulous treatment of hypertension (also important in preventing progression of CRF)
- A lower threshold for preventive measures (antiplatelet agents, lipid-lowering drugs and folic acid) may be appropriate, but this is not proved. Potentially these interventions could also influence the progression of CRF (based on animal studies). Human studies are in progress (e.g. the Heart and Renal Protection study).

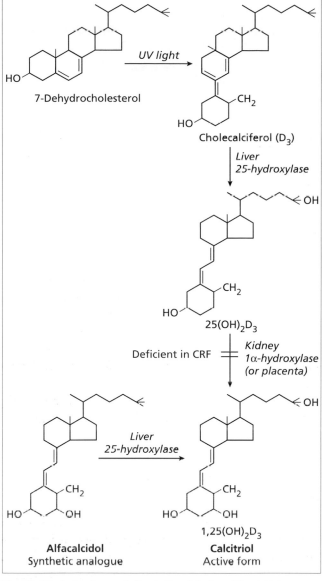

Fig. 44 Principal pathway of vitamin D metabolism. Alfacalcidol or calcitriol are used to treat patients with renal impairment.

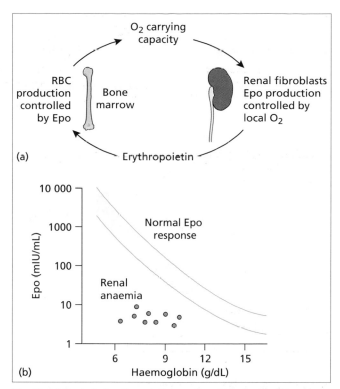

Fig. 45 (a) Control of erythropoietin secretion. (b) Patients with renal impairment (red dots) have a relative deficiency in erythropoietin secretion, with reduced levels of circulating erythropoietin compared to the normal response for a given level of haemoglobin.

with chronic renal impairment, pregnancy results in additional deterioration in renal function superimposed on the predicted course of their chronic renal impairment.

The chance of successful fetal outcome and risk to maternal renal function can be stratified on the basis of renal impairment, hypertension and proteinuria. Normal pregnancy is rare with creatinine >275 μmol/L. See Section 1.2 for further discussion.

Drugs

Dose adjustments are required for many medications. Take care to avoid nephrotoxic drugs. If in doubt look in the BNF.

Preparation for renal replacement therapy

Once it is clear that the patient will develop end-stage renal failure, preparation for renal replacement therapy should be made well in advance (e.g. formation of arteriovenous fistula for haemodialysis).

Prognosis

The effect of chronic renal impairment on morbidity and mortality is uncertain. The tendency to progress correlates closely with the following:

Gout

Gout is common. Reduced urate excretion and diuretics are the major factors. It is often confused with pseudogout (pyrophosphate). Generally treat acute episodes with colchicine (avoiding NSAIDs). Prevention with allopurinol (if urate high or after an episode).

 Remember to reduce the dose of allopurinol in renal impairment.

Pregnancy in chronic renal impairment

As renal function declines, the ability to conceive and to carry a pregnancy successfully declines. In some women

- The amount of proteinuria
- The amount of interstitial damage on the renal biopsy
- Higher in men than in women.

The likelihood of end-stage renal failure obviously increases as functional reserve decreases. The most useful guide is the trend in GFR.

> 1 Klahr S, Levey AS, Beck GJ *et al*. The effects of dietary protein restriction and blood-pressure control on the progression of chronic renal disease. *N Engl J Med* 1994; 330: 877–884.
> 2 Lewis EJ, Hunsicker LG, Bain RP, Rohde RD. The effect of angiotensin-converting enzyme inhibition on diabetic nephropathy. *N Engl J Med* 1993; 329: 1456–1462.

2.1.3 END-STAGE RENAL FAILURE

End-stage renal failure is the point at which renal function is no longer sufficient for normal life as a result of irreversible loss of renal function, i.e. the point at which renal replacement therapy should be commenced (if appropriate for the patient).

Aetiology/pathophysiology/pathology

At a certain level of GFR, accumulation of molecules that are usually excreted by the kidney reaches a level at which they prevent or endanger normal physiological functions. The principal problems are:

- Potassium
- Salt and water
- Hydrogen ions
- Uraemic toxins.

The term 'uraemic toxins' refers to the vast numbers of chemicals that accumulate in the blood as the kidneys fail. Urea and creatinine are the two measured in clinical practice, but do not correlate very strongly with uraemic symptoms (those made better by dialysis). Elderly people and those with less muscle mass will have a lower GFR for any given creatinine, and will reach end-stage renal failure with a lower creatinine (e.g. 450 vs 850 µmol/L).

> As patients approach end-stage renal failure, they frequently become malnourished because of loss of appetite, resulting in muscle wasting and deceptively low creatinine. The correct treatment is dialysis and attention to nutrition.

Epidemiology

The take-on rate for renal replacement therapy in the UK is approximately 92/million population per year. End-stage renal failure is much more common in elderly than in young people (Fig. 46). Causes are as for CRF.

Clinical presentation

Symptoms are sensitive, but not very specific:
- Tiredness, difficulty concentrating
- Loss of appetite
- Nausea and vomiting.

If these are present in a patient with a creatinine above 450 µmol/L, serious consideration should be given to commencing dialysis unless there is another cause (e.g. anaemia contributing to tiredness). In severe cases, presentation may be with pericarditis, uraemic encephalopathy or neuropathy. In others, the need for dialysis will be precipitated by acidosis, hyperkalaemia or fluid overload resistant to diuretics and sodium restriction.

> Monitoring patients with renal impairment as they approach end-stage renal failure should allow them to be commenced on dialysis at a time when symptoms are minimal, but they will feel a clear benefit.

> Early referral to a renal unit allows emphasis to be placed on delaying progression of end-stage renal failure, avoiding complications, and physical and psychological preparations for renal replacement therapy.

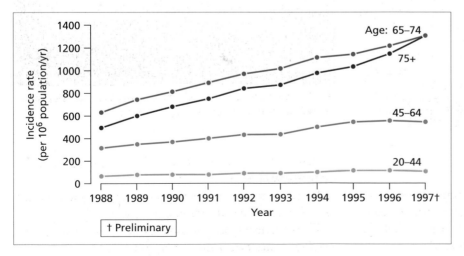

Fig. 46 Take-on rate for renal replacement therapy according to age in the USA (data from the United States Renal Data System annual report, 1999). The increase in the older population is mainly due to increased willingness to dialyse these patients. Similar trends are observed in the UK and Europe.

Physical signs

• Commonly, there are no physical signs when a patient reaches end-stage renal failure
• Less commonly, pericardial rub or metabolic flap may be present
• Peripheral neuropathy, uraemic frost and fits are rare.

Investigations

• Identify the cause of the renal damage if possible (as for CRF).
• Establish that the diagnosis is CRF: small kidneys on ultrasonography; evidence of previous renal impairment. If kidneys are normal size and not obstructed, a renal biopsy will usually be indicated.
• Consider whether there is a reversible factor causing acute-on-chronic renal failure: volume depletion or hypotension, nephrotoxic drugs (e.g. NSAIDs), prostatic obstruction.
• Test for hepatitis B and C: potentially infectious patients will require special dialysis arrangements. Others should be immunized against hepatitis B.

Treatment

• Commence renal replacement therapy—if the need is urgent, haemodialysis will usually be used initially
• If there is cardiovascular instability, haemofiltration may be preferred to begin with
• Emergency treatment for hyperkalaemia (see Section 1.6, pp. 16–20) may be indicated pending transfer for dialysis.

 It is unwise to defer dialysis—if in doubt, dialyse first and ask questions later.

It is important to appreciate that dialysis is equivalent only to a low level of GFR—in the region of 6 mL/min. Although sometimes patients (and occasionally their doctors) will suggest dialysis in the context of less severe renal impairment, this would represent a relatively small increment in clearance compared with the patient's own renal function. This is unlikely to lead to clinical benefit, would be at considerable financial cost, and would also be a major inconvenience to the patient.

Complications

These are as listed for chronic renal impairment (Section 2.1.2, pp. 50–56). The following are particular problems in patients with end-stage renal disease treated by dialysis:
• Increased cardiovascular mortality (Fig. 47)

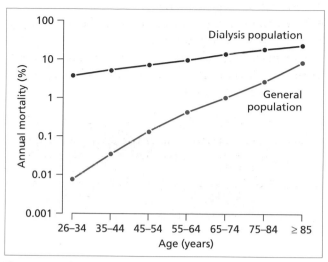

Fig. 47 Annual mortality in the general population and dialysis patients (data from the United States Renal Data System 1994–96). Mortality is increased over 100-fold in younger dialysis patients.

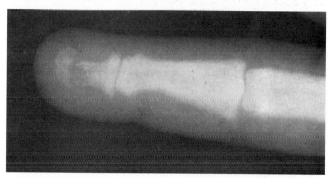

Fig. 48 Radiograph of the finger of a haemodialysis patient with severe hyperparathyroidism. There is subperiosteal resorption and osteo-acrolysis.

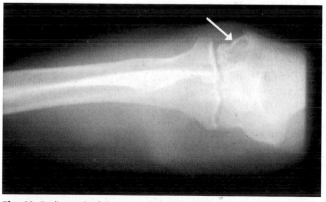

Fig. 49 Radiograph of the wrist of a longstanding haemodialysis patient. The radiolucent area (arrow) is an amyloid deposit.

• Autonomous hyperparathyroidism, requiring parathyroidectomy (Fig. 48)
• Accumulation of β_2-microglobulin amyloid with carpal tunnel syndrome and arthropathy (Fig. 49).

There are also specific complications of the renal replacement therapies (see Section 2.2, pp. 61–72).

Prognosis

In appropriate patients dialysis can usually be performed relatively smoothly and safely, especially when adequate practical and psychological preparation is made.

On renal replacement therapy, mortality is much higher than in a population matched for age, diabetes, etc. (Fig. 47).

Prevention

• Measures to prevent progression of CRF (see Section 2.1.2, pp. 50–56)
• If there is sufficient advance planning, transplantation before end-stage renal failure is reached—either from a living or cadaveric donor—may avoid the need for dialysis.

http://www.usrds.org—The US Renal Data System (USRDS) national data system collects, analyses and distributes information about end-stage renal disease.
http://www.renalreg.com—The UK Renal Registry is undertaking a similar function in the UK.

2.1.4 NEPHROTIC SYNDROME

Nephrotic syndrome is the combination of:
• Proteinuria (usually >3.0 g/24 h)
• Hypoalbuminaemia (<35 g/L)
• Oedema.

Aetiology/pathophysiology/pathology

Proteinuria

The underlying defect is increased glomerular permeability to protein. Some of the leaked protein is absorbed and catabolized by the tubular cells; the remainder is passed in the urine. The normal glomerulus selects which molecules can pass from the circulation to the tubular space based on:
• size
• electrical charge.
  Size selectivity relates to:
• fenestrae in the endothelium
• pores in the basement membrane
• slit diaphragms between the foot processes of the epithelial cells (podocytes).

Charge selectivity is the result of electrostatic repulsion of negatively charged proteins by negative charge on the basement membrane and endothelium.

In some patients with congenital nephrotic syndrome a recently identified protein, nephrin, is absent from the slit diaphragm. In other settings the precise mechanism(s) resulting in substantial filtration of protein is not well understood, although it is clear that there is altered size

selectivity, usually allowing passage of considerable amounts of IgG (radius about 5.5 nm) in addition to albumin. There is also reduced charge selectivity. Classification of causes of the nephrotic syndrome is by histological appearance: some have specific treatments.

Hypoalbuminaemia

The circulating albumin concentration does not correlate tightly with the proteinuria as a result of the variable extent of tubular catabolism. The amount of compensatory increase in hepatic synthesis is also variable.

Oedema

An attractive hypothesis was that the oedema is driven by hypovolaemia caused by reduced plasma oncotic pressure, resulting in compensatory sodium retention.

This simple explanation cannot be sustained in adults, although may apply in children with minimal change disease. Plasma volume is not reduced in untreated sodium-retaining adult nephritis; sodium retention does not correlate well with renin–angiotensin activation; and converting enzyme inhibitors are not natriuretic.

Epidemiology

Underlying histological diagnosis varies with age (Fig. 50). Not included are large numbers of people with diabetes who are technically late in the course of diabetic nephropathy, but in whom a renal biopsy would not be appropriate.

Most children with nephrotic syndrome are steroid responsive (minimal change nephrotic syndrome or focal segmental glomerulosclerosis [FSGS]). Under the age of 10, it is therefore usual to treat with steroids and only biopsy non-responders.

Clinical presentation

• Usually with peripheral oedema
• May be of gradual or sudden onset
• Ranges from trivial to a major problem resistant to diuretics, etc.
• Some children present with abrupt onset of massive proteinuria, hypovolaemia and even collapse
• Elderly patients with minimal change nephrotic syndrome may present with acute renal failure
• Sometimes the patient will notice frothy urine (Fig. 51).

Investigations

Investigations aim to do the following:
• Confirm that the patient is nephrotic
• Assess the severity of the protein leak

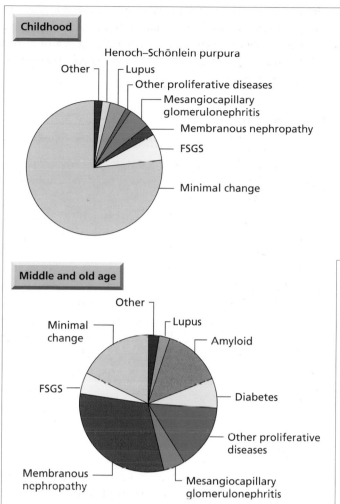

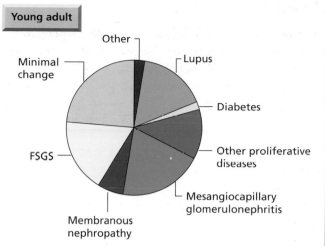

Fig. 50 Histological diagnoses of renal biopsies of 1000 patients at Guy's Hospital from 1963–90. (Redrawn from J.S.Cameron In: A.M. Davison *et al* (eds) *Oxford Textbook of Clinical Nephrology*, 2nd edn, Oxford: Oxford University Press, 1998).

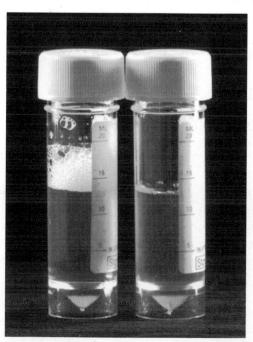

Fig. 51 Urine from a nephrotic patient with a protein content of 5 g/L (left) and a normal sample (right).

- Obtain a histological diagnosis of the glomerular abnormality.

Investigations should include the following:
- Serum albumin and creatinine
- Urinalysis and microscopy: presence of some red cells does not rule out minimal change, but makes it less likely
- 24-h collection to estimate protein excretion, or spot protein/creatinine ratio (see Section 3.1, pp. 106–107)
- Renal ultrasonography: scars suggest reflux nephropathy; if single kidney, biopsy would not normally be performed
- Chest radiograph
- Protein electrophoresis: urine and serum.

Other investigations could be refined on the basis of the histological diagnosis and/or other clinical information, the following being examples:
- Systemic lupus erythematosus (SLE) gives positive ANF and low complement levels
- Hepatitis B is associated with membranous nephropathy
- Hepatitis C is associated with cryoglobulinaemia and mesangiocapillary glomerulonephritis (MCGN).

Adults (and children over the age of 10) will almost always have a renal biopsy.

Differential diagnosis

• Oedema commonly results from other factors (e.g. congestive cardiac failure [CCF])
• Proteinuria: dipstick testing of the urine is very sensitive, and minor proteinuria occurs in many situations (e.g. CCF, fever)
• Hypoalbuminaemia is common in other circumstances (liver disease, chronic illness).

Treatment

Oedema

The success of symptomatic treatment is best monitored by daily weighing; aim to reduce by 0.5–1.0 kg/day.

To achieve negative sodium balance, do the following:
• Restrict dietary sodium.
• Diuretics will almost always be necessary, usually furosemide (frusemide)/bumetanide. Large doses are often required (partly because bound by filtered protein in the tubular lumen). In resistant cases, additional diuretics that act synergistically, e.g. metolazone, may be needed, also potassium supplements and/or amiloride.
• Severe cases may be treated with the combination of intravenous 20% albumin and diuretics, or haemofiltration.

Reduction of proteinuria

• Where appropriate the underlying process is treated, e.g. steroids in minimal change.
• ACE inhibitors reduce proteinuria and slow deterioration in GFR. Use may be restricted by hypotension.
• Refractory cases: NSAIDs or cyclosporin are sometimes used to reduce proteinuria in refractory cases. The effect results mainly from a reduction in GFR. Such cases should be distinguished from the use of cyclosporin to treat the underlying condition (relapsing minimal change or membranous glomerulonephritis). Nephrectomy and renal replacement therapy are rarely justified in exceptional cases of refractory oedema.

Complications

Hyperlipidaemia

Over half of nephrotic patients have cholesterol >7.5 mmol/L.
• High-density lipoprotein (HDL) often decreased
• Low-density lipoprotein (LDL) synthesis is increased and catabolism decreased.

It is not clear what impact this has on cardiovascular risk, but concern is obviously increased with increased duration of nephrotic syndrome. HMG-CoA reductase inhibitors do lower cholesterol in this group and are considered on the basis of the overall risk profile (see Section 1.4, pp. 10–13).

Thrombosis

10–40% of patients with the nephrotic syndrome develop deep venous thrombosis (DVT) or renal vein thrombosis (Fig. 52). This is probably less common in minimal change nephrotic syndrome. Prothrombotic abnormalities include reduced antithrombin III (urinary losses). Renal vein thrombosis may present with:
• pulmonary emboli (Fig. 53)
• decrease in GFR
• flank pain and haematuria.

Diagnosed on selective venography, venous phase of renal angiogram (see Fig. 52), computed tomography or magnetic resonance imaging.

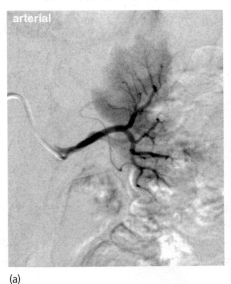

(a)

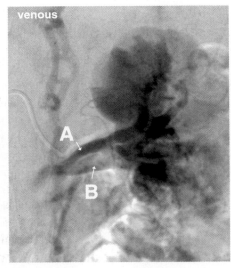

(b)

Fig. 52 Digital subtraction angiography in a patient with membranous nephropathy. On the venous phase (b) there is defective filling of the inferior renal vein (B). The superior renal vein (A) fills normally.

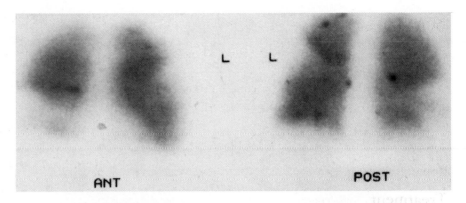
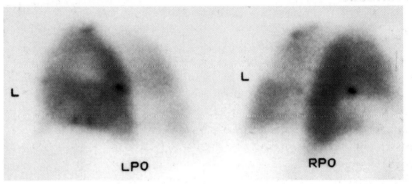

Fig. 53 Lung perfusion scan of the same patient as Fig. 52 showing multiple defects consistent with pulmonary emboli.

Prevention

• Primary prevention: oral anticoagulants may be considered in ambulant patients with severe nephrotic syndrome
• Secondary prevention: after an episode of thrombosis anticoagulation should continue as long as the patient remains nephrotic.

Infections

• Primary peritonitis (usually with *Streptococcus pneumoniae*) can occur in children. Low concentrations of complement factor B (55 kDa), which is necessary for alternative pathway activation, might explain this propensity. Most adults are probably protected by antibodies to capsular antigens. Consider prophylactic penicillin in children.
• Cellulitis is frequent, presumably as a result of immunological factors and skin fragility/oedema.

Deterioration in renal function

Minimal change nephrotic syndrome does not lead to chronic deterioration in renal function. Other histological categories carry a substantial risk of progressive loss of GFR, which varies according to histological diagnosis (see Section 2.3, pp. 72–80).

Prognosis

This varies with the histological diagnosis (see Section 2.3, pp. 72–80).

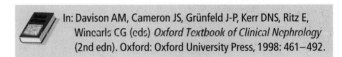

In: Davison AM, Cameron JS, Grünfeld J-P, Kerr DNS, Ritz E, Winearls CG (eds) *Oxford Textbook of Clinical Nephrology* (2nd edn). Oxford: Oxford University Press, 1998: 461–492.

2.2 Renal replacement therapy

The following modalities are available:
• Haemodialysis
• Peritoneal dialysis
• Transplantation.

The main advantage of transplantation is that it can effectively restore normal renal function. However, it requires a major operation and immunosuppression, and is unsuccessful in a proportion of cases. Transplantation is also restricted by the availability of donor organs.

The relative pros and cons of haemodialysis and peritoneal dialysis are outlined in Table 18.

2.2.1 HAEMODIALYSIS

Principle

Haemodialysis involves circulating the patient's blood, via some form of vascular access (Table 19), through an extracorporeal circulation where it is exposed to an isotonic buffered dialysis solution across a semipermeable membrane.

	Advantages	Disadvantages
Haemodialysis*	• Hospital based treatment offers feeling of safety with responsibility resting with renal staff • Intermittent sessions offer an escape from treatment for much of the week • Dialysis isn't brought into the home environment	• Regular journeys to and from hospital • Involves regular use of needles • Long treatment sessions attached to a machine away from home • More stringent dietary and fluid restrictions due to intermittent nature of treatment • More restrictive on travel
Home haemodialysis	• Flexibility • Much less frequent journeys to the hospital • Treatment in a more comfortable environment (home)	• Needs extensive training • Requires conversion of a room at home • Brings dialysis into the patient's home life
Peritoneal dialysis†	• In control of own treatment • Less frequent visits to hospital • Easy to travel and holiday abroad • Can be integrated into most jobs	• Not always suitable for patients with no residual function or large muscle mass • Peritonitis • Technique survival beyond 5–10 years is not well established

Table 18 Advantages and disadvantages of different dialysis modalities.

*See Section 2.2.1, pp. 61–65.
†See Section 2.2.2, pp. 65–69.

Table 19 Haemodialysis vascular access.

Temporary dialysis catheter (Fig. 54)	Principally for acute temporary dialysis. Large-bore dual lumen polythene catheters. Inserted into femoral, internal jugular or subclavian veins. The subclavian route carries a risk of vein stenosis making AV fistula formation on that side less successful
Semi-Permanent dialysis catheter (Fig. 55)	Large-bore dual lumen silicone catheters for medium-term use, i.e. months. Usually inserted into the internal jugular veins and tunnelled subcutaneously to an exit point high on the chest wall. A dacron cuff provides stability and reduces infection rates
AV fistula (Fig. 56)	The optimum long-term access. Made by anastamosing the radial or brachial artery to a vein. Take 1–4 months to mature. Can last >10 years. No foreign material so infection risk is very low. Success depends on good native vessels
PTFE grafts	If native veins unsuitable for anastamosis to an artery then a graft can be used. Either straight grafts (e.g. brachial artery to axillary vein) or as a loop. Can usually be used within 2 weeks. Life span limited to a few years. Infection, when it occurs, is a major problem

PTFE, polytetrafluoroethylene.

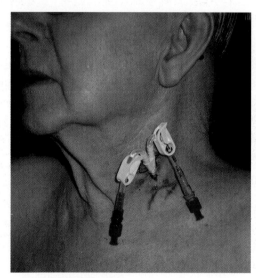

Fig. 54 Temporary dialysis line inserted in the left internal jugular vein.

Toxin removal

This occurs through diffusion. Waste products are at high concentration in the patient's blood but absent from the buffered dialysis solution. Diffusion involves the passage of these toxins down this concentration gradient (Fig. 57).

Fluid removal

This occurs through ultrafiltration. Water moves down a pressure gradient across the dialysis membrane from the blood into the dialysis solution (Fig. 58). Modern dialysis machines regulate removal of fluid by regulating this transmembrane pressure (TMP). Some solute molecules move with the water by convection.

Indications

Acute and chronic renal failure: issues affecting when to initiate dialysis are discussed in Section 2.1 (pp. 48–61) and Table 9.

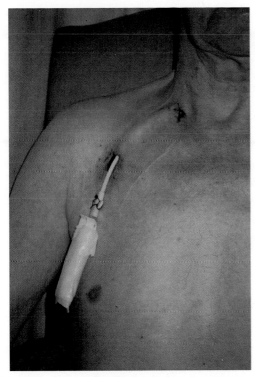

Fig. 55 Semi-permanent dialysis line inserted into the right internal jugular vein.

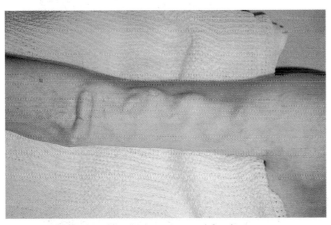

Fig. 56 Well developed brachial arteriovenous fistula.

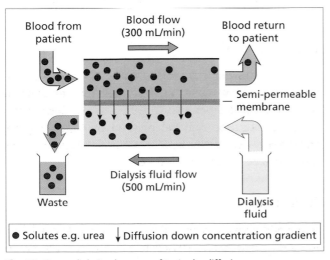

Blood from patient

Blood flow (300 mL/min)

Blood return to patient

Semi-permeable membrane

Dialysis fluid flow (500 mL/min)

Waste

Dialysis fluid

● Solutes e.g. urea ↓ Diffusion down concentration gradient

Fig. 57 Haemodialysis: clearance of toxins by diffusion.

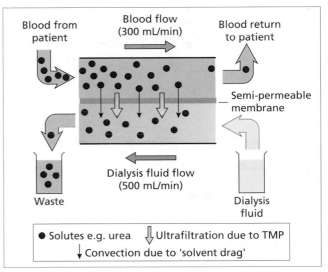

Blood from patient

Blood flow (300 mL/min)

Blood return to patient

Semi-permeable membrane

Dialysis fluid flow (500 mL/min)

Waste

Dialysis fluid

● Solutes e.g. urea ⇩ Ultrafiltration due to TMP
↓ Convection due to 'solvent drag'

Fig. 58 Haemodialysis: ultrafiltration (fluid removal) is driven by the transmembrane pressure (TMP) across the semi-permeable membrane.

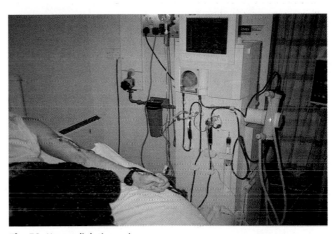

Fig. 59 Haemodialysis session.

 Do not wait for the development of an urgent indication for dialysis before referring or starting treatment.
Prepare well in advance. The need for good vascular access together with adequate information and education necessitates early planning. Most units would start this at least 1 year before the predicted need for dialysis.

Contraindications

Patients with severe cardiovascular compromise may not tolerate either the extracorporeal circuit or fluid removal.

Practical details

The machinery and circuit for haemodialysis are illustrated in Figs 59 and 60. Most patients in the UK receive three 4-h treatments a week.

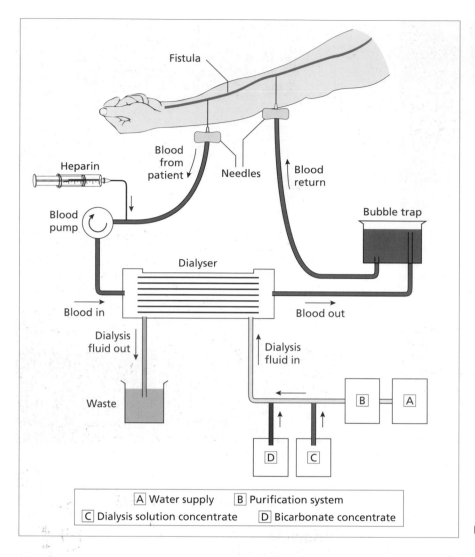

A Water supply   B Purification system
C Dialysis solution concentrate   D Bicarbonate concentrate

Fig. 60 Basic haemodialysis circuit.

Dialysis treatment parameters

- Target weight or amount of fluid to be removed: assess volume status off dialysis. Set a target and reassess.
- Type and size of dialysis membrane: larger membrane surface area gives more dialysis. High-flux membranes clear middle molecules such as β_2-microglobulin with greater efficiency. Biocompatible membranes cause less activation of inflammatory pathways in the patient and may be advantageous in some settings.
- Time on dialysis.
- Type of dialysis fluid: parameters adjusted are sodium, potassium, bicarbonate and calcium.
- Anticoagulation: heparin dose.

Dialysis adequacy

There is evidence for a threshold amount of dialysis below which morbidity and mortality increase. There are national targets for measured dialysis adequacy. Increasing the amount of dialysis delivered requires either:

- an increase in the weekly time on dialysis, or
- greater dialysis efficiency.

Complications

The following are common complications:
- Hypotension on dialysis
- Bacteraemia
- Problems related to vascular access (Table 20).

Hypotension

The following are the main causes of hypotension during haemodialysis:

- Incorrect target weight: too much fluid removed, leading to absolute volume depletion
- Rate of fluid removal too high: not enough time for refilling of vascular compartment from interstitial compartment
- Poor compensatory response to volume removal: this is common in autonomic neuropathy associated with diabetes.

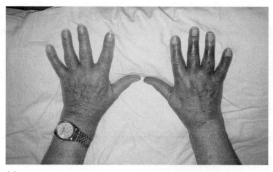
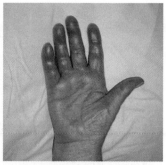

Fig. 61 Dusky ischaemic right hand secondary to vascular steal by forearm dialysis fistula.

(a)

(b)

Table 20 Problems related to vascular access.

Infection	Common, often involves multiresistant organisms. Temporary (non-tunnelled) venous catheters carry the highest risk. Once infected it is rarely possible to sterilize prosthetic material
Blockage, thrombosis or poor flow rates	Multiple factors including hypotension, increased blood viscosity, vessel stenoses, line-associated fibrin sheath. For lines can try urokinase. For grafts and fistula possibilities include thrombolysis, surgical revision or angioplasty. Prophylaxis with warfarin or dipyridamole may help
Vascular steal syndromes	Mainly a complication of arteriovenous fistulas (Fig. 61). Pain is worse during dialysis. Usually need to be tied off
High-output cardiac failure	Very uncommon

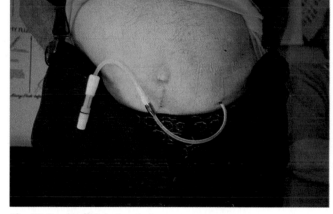

Fig. 62 Tenckhoff dialysis catheter.

2.2.2 PERITONEAL DIALYSIS

Principle

As with haemodialysis, peritoneal dialysis exposes the patient's blood to a buffered dialysis solution across a semipermeable membrane. However, the blood remains in the body and the semipermeable membrane is the peritoneum. Dialysis fluid is introduced via a silicone catheter (Fig. 62).

Toxin removal

This occurs through diffusion and convection. Small molecules diffuse across the peritoneal membrane down the concentration gradient between the blood and intraperitoneal dialysis solution (Fig. 63). Larger molecules tend to move through convection or solvent drag associated with the movement of fluid.

Fluid removal (ultrafiltration)

This occurs through osmosis. Water moves across the semipermeable membrane to equilibrate the osmolalities of the two compartments (Fig. 63). Peritoneal dialysis solutions are manufactured to be hyperosmolar. Dextrose is the usual osmotic agent: use of different concentrations (1.36%, 2.27% or 3.6%) allows control of fluid removal.

> **Prevention of haemodialysis-related hypotension**
>
> - Reset target weight
> - Reduce rate of fluid removal: either more frequent dialysis or longer session
> - Sodium profiling: increasing the [Na⁺] of dialysis fluid early in the session reduces osmotic shifts in the patient that tend to cause volume contraction; the downside is sodium loading and increased thirst
> - Cool dialysis fluid—causes vasoconstriction
> - Omit antihypertensives on dialysis day.

Important information for patients

Haemodialysis puts the patient in an unfamiliar, complex and frequently frightening environment. Appropriate information and support are essential and best handled by an integrated team, including specialist nurses, doctors, dietitians and psychologists.

Maher JF, ed. *Replacement of Renal Function by Dialysis.* Dordrecht: Kluwer Academic Publishers Group, 1989
http://www.kidney.org/professionals/doqi/doqi/index.html.

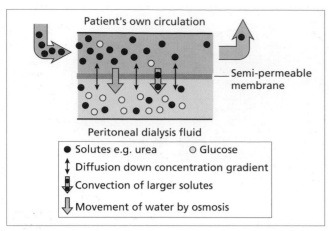

Fig. 63 Mechanisms underlying peritoneal dialysis.

Peritoneal transport characteristics

The rate at which solutes cross the peritoneal membrane varies in different individuals (Fig. 64):
• Low transporters: require long dwell times to reach maximum toxin clearance. Most suited to continuous ambulatory peritoneal dialysis (CAPD).
• High transporters: rapidly remove toxins, even with short dwell times. Rapidly absorb dextrose, thus losing the osmotic gradient with associated poor ultrafiltration. Best suited to automated peritoneal dialysis (APD).

Indications

Long-term maintenance renal replacement therapy.

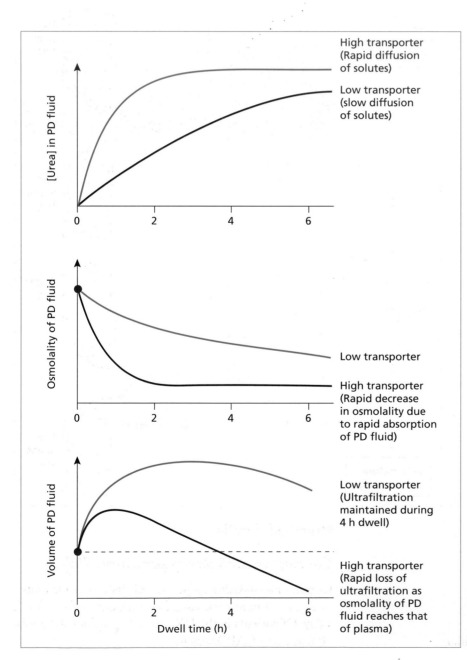

Fig. 64 Solute transport properties of the peritoneal membrane. High transporters rapidly clear toxins by diffusion, but also quickly experience a fall in dialysis fluid osmolality as a result of rapid uptake of glucose, which leads to poor ultrafiltration. Low transporters take longer to clear toxins by diffusion but ultrafiltration is good because glucose uptake from the dialysis fluid is slower.

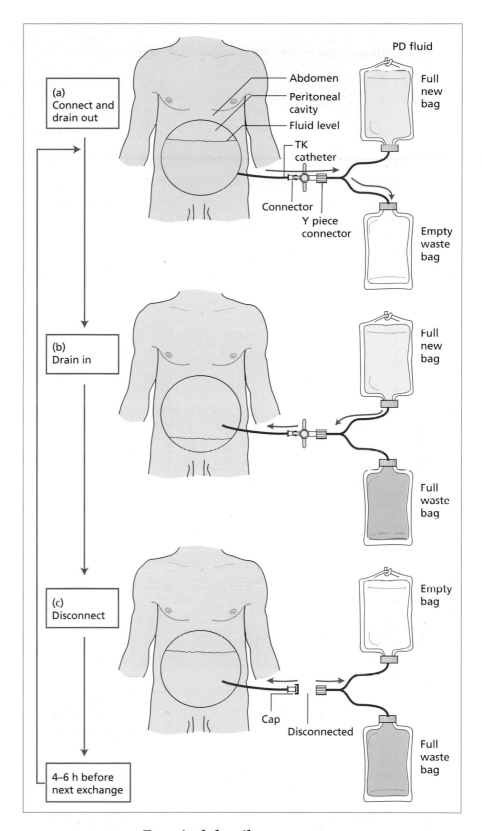

Fig. 65 Continuous ambulatory peritoneal dialysis (CAPD): (a) a Y connector with an empty waste bag and a bag with fresh dialysis fluid is attached to the Tenckhoff (TK) catheter. Dialysis fluid is drained into the waste bag. (b) The Y connector is switched to drain in the fresh dialysis fluid. (c) The Y connector is removed. The patient is now free for 4–6 h.

Contraindications

Most are relative:
- Previous major abdominal surgery
- Diverticulitis
- Hernia
- Chronic respiratory disease
- Unable to learn and perform technique.

Practical details

Continuous ambulatory peritoneal dialysis

Continuous ambulatory peritoneal dialysis is illustrated in Fig. 65. There are usually four exchanges of 1.5–3.0 L a day. Of patients in the UK receiving peritoneal dialysis, 90% are on a CAPD system.

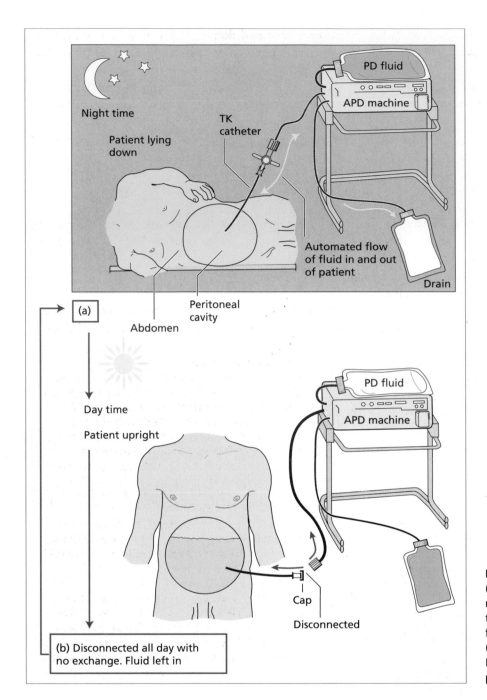

Fig. 66 Automated peritoneal dialysis (APD): (a) at bedtime the patient connects to the machine with sufficient dialysis solution for the night. The machine delivers and drains fluid automatically throughout the night. (b) In the morning the patient disconnects. Fluid is left inside the peritoneal cavity. The patient is now free until bedtime.

Night time

Patient lying down

PD fluid

APD machine

TK catheter

Automated flow of fluid in and out of patient

Drain

(a)

Abdomen

Peritoneal cavity

Day time

Patient upright

PD fluid

APD machine

Cap

Disconnected

(b) Disconnected all day with no exchange. Fluid left in

Automated peritoneal dialysis

Automated peritoneal dialysis (APD) is illustrated in Fig. 66. Only 10% of UK patients use APD, although this is increasing. The patient is free from day-time exchanges. The usual regimen (continuous cyclic peritoneal dialysis or CCPD) involves four or five cycles overnight of 2–2.5 L each with short dwell times. After the last cycle, fluid is left in until the next evening.

Dialysis adequacy

The clearance on peritoneal dialysis can be measured: below a minimum level mortality appears to be increased [1].

- Increasing the amount of dialysis in CAPD is usually limited to five exchanges per day of 2.5- to 3-L bags. Over time, as residual renal function reduces, many patients cannot achieve adequate dialysis with CAPD.
- Some will succeed with the APD system, but most need to switch to haemodialysis.

Outcome

Compared with haemodialysis, patient survival on peritoneal dialysis is probably equivalent after correction for co-morbidity and age. Technique survival is inferior to that for haemodialysis. The following factors are involved:

- Ultrafiltration failure: as a result of either increased

peritoneal membrane permeability or membrane sclerosis. The first group can convert to APD but the second need haemodialysis.
• Recurrent peritonitis.
• Inability to increase dialysis to adequate levels as residual function declines.

Complications

• Peritonitis: the greatest problem associated with peritoneal dialysis. Often associated with exit site infection or poor technique. Presentation is with abdominal pain and/or cloudy dialysate. Diagnosis is suggested by finding >100 cells/mm^3 and >50% neutrophils in the peritoneal dialysate. Treatment involves antibiotics, often given in the dialysis fluid. Failure to respond or recurrent peritonitis often requires catheter removal.
• Poor dialysis fluid drainage: factors include constipation and/or malpositioned catheter.
• Physical problems: hernias are relatively common. Leakage of fluid can occur at the exit site, through the diaphragm causing a pleural effusion, or into the abdominal wall or the perineal area. May require a new catheter or change to haemodialysis.
• Sclerosing peritonitis: rare and sometimes fatal.

Important information for patients

Peritoneal dialysis requires education, training and ongoing support. Usually the key figure is a specialist nurse.

Maher JF, ed. *Replacement of Renal Function by Dialysis.* Dordrecht: Kluwer Academic Publishers Group, 1989.
Gentil MA, Carriazo A, Pavon MI *et al.* Comparison of survival in continuous ambulatory peritoneal dialysis and hospital haemodialysis: a multicentric study. *Nephrol Dial Transplant* 1991; 6: 444–451.
Churchil DN, Thorp KE, Nolph KD, Keshaviah PR, Oreopoulos DG, Page D. Increased peritoneal membrane transport is associated with decreased patient and technique survival for continuous peritoneal dialysis patients. The Canada–USA (CANUSA) Peritoneal Dialysis Study Group. *J Am Soc Nephrol* 1998; 9: 1285–1292.
1 http://www.kidney.org/professionals/doqi/doqi/index.html

2.2.3 RENAL TRANSPLANTATION

Principle

The principle is to implant a functioning healthy kidney and prevent rejection by the immune system.

Source of kidneys

• Living related donors: sibling to sibling and parent to child are the most common pairings.

• Living unrelated donors: this is relatively uncommon in the UK, but donation by a spouse/partner is becoming more common.
• Cadaveric: heart-beating donors who satisfy the criteria of brain death. This is the main source of organs in the UK.
• Cadaveric: non-heart beating donors. Limited to a few UK centres. Results are less good with a high rate of delayed or non-function.

Indications

In most patients requiring renal replacement therapy, the possibility of kidney transplantation should be considered.

Contraindications

A range of issues affects suitability for transplantation and the overall likelihood of benefit compared with dialysis.

Patient survival issues
• Malignancy: there is a significant risk of recurrence even after apparent curative treatment; waiting at least 2–3 years before considering transplantation may reduce this risk
• Cardiovascular disease: patients with coronary artery disease (which may be asymptomatic and is frequent in patients with end-stage renal failure) have a high early postoperative mortality; this may be reduced by intervention before transplantation.

Graft survival issues
• Patient survival: patient death is one of the commonest causes of graft loss, so patient survival issues are important
• Previous renal disease: the original disease process should be considered; FSGS and MCGN carry significant risks of recurrence and graft loss
• Efficient and equitable resource allocation: successful transplantation becomes more cost-effective than dialysis after about 2 years. There is a balance between maximizing the potential of each graft in terms of patient-years off dialysis and the benefit to individual patients of a graft lasting as long as they live, even if that is fairly short.

Practical details

The waiting list

Potential cadaveric transplant recipients are enrolled onto the UK register which is managed by the UK Transplant Support Service Authority. The patient's tissue type (HLA-A, -B and -DR) is determined and blood is screened for cytotoxic antibodies. HIV testing is required.

Call-up for a potential transplant

Allocation from the national pool is on a points system (HLA matching, donor/recipient relative age, time on waiting list, etc.). Preoperatively, recipient serum and donor

Drug	Mode of action	Use	Common problems
Prednisolone	Multiple effects on inflammatory and immunological pathways	Maintenance Acute rejection (methylprednisolone)	Osteoporosis Avascular necrosis Diabetogenic Weight gain Dyslipidaemia Hypertension Peptic ulceration Cataracts
Azathioprine	Blocks purine synthesis and hence cell proliferation	Maintenance	Bone marrow suppression
Cyclosporin	Calcineurin inhibitor; blocks intracellular signals involved in T-cell activation	Maintenance	Nephrotoxicity Hypertension CNS toxicity especially tremor Hirsuitism Gum hypertrophy Diabetogenic
Tacrolimus	Calcineurin inhibitor; blocks intracellular signals involved in T-cell activation	Maintenance	Nephrotoxicity Hypertension Diabetogenic CNS toxicity especially tremor
Mycophenolate mofetil	Blocks purine synthesis in lymphocytes by inhibiting inosine monophosphate dehydrogenase	Maintenance	Diarrhoea Bone marrow suppression
Sirolimus	Blocks intracellular signals involved in T-cell activation and impairs cytokine signalling		Thrombocytopaenia Leucopaenia Hypercholesterolaemia
Antithymocyte globulin (ATG)	Direct T-cell lysis. Other cell types are affected as it is a polyclonal preparation	Induction and acute rejection	Fever Increased rate of PTLD
OKT3	Direct T-cell lysis through CD3-activation-induced cell death	Induction and acute rejection	Cytokine release syndrome Increased rate of PTLD
Basiliximab	Anti IL2 receptor antibody; prevents IL2-dependent T-cell proliferation and activation	Induction	Immunosuppression
Daclizumab	Blocks tac subunit of IL2 receptor; prevents IL2-dependent T-cell proliferation and activation	Induction	Anaphylaxis Immunosuppression

Table 21 Immunosuppressive drugs used in renal transplantation. For further information see *Immunology and immunosuppression*, Section 8.

PTLD, post-transplant lymphoproliferative disorder.

lymphocytes are crossmatched to detect preformed antibodies that would preclude transplantation in cases where there is a risk of this happening.

The operation

The kidney is placed extraperitoneally in the iliac fossa and vessels anastomosed, usually to the external iliac artery and vein. The ureter is implanted into the bladder.

Immunosuppression

Individual drugs are detailed in Table 21. Various regimens are used. Most use a combination of a calineurin inhibitor + steroids ± azathioprine. After about 4 weeks of stable graft function, doses are gradually reduced, reaching maintenance levels by about 6 months.

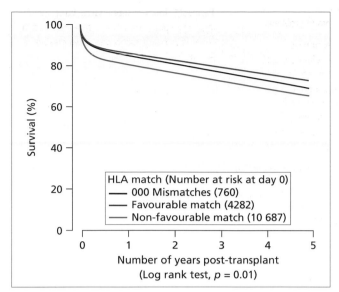

Fig. 67 Transplant survival for UK first cadaveric kidney grafts, 1990–97, stratified by HLA mismatches. (Reproduced with permission from UK Transplant Support Service Authority.)

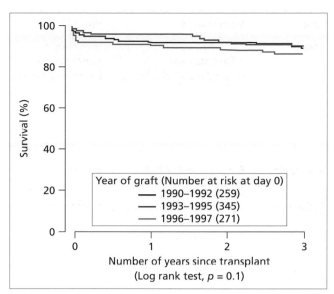

Fig. 68 Transplant survival for UK adult live donor kidney grafts, 1990–97, stratified by year of grafting. (Reproduced with permission from UK Transplant Support Service Authority.)

Other therapies

- Aspirin: may reduce risk of renal vein thrombosis
- Calcium channel blockers: may reduce calineurin inhibitor toxicity
- Co-trimoxazole prophylaxis against *Pneumocystis carinii* pneumonia (PCP).

Unless long-term indications exist, these are usually discontinued by 3 months after transplantation.

Outcome

The UK 5-year graft survival rate for first cadaveric transplantation is 63.9–71.4% depending on the degree of HLA matching (Fig. 67). The UK 3-year survival rate for live related grafts is just under 90% (Fig. 68).

Comparison of patients who are transplanted with those on the transplant waiting list demonstrates a longer-term survival benefit from transplantation, although there is an initial increase in mortality for the first year. Relative to staying on dialysis, patients with diabetes benefit the most, although absolute survival is less. Extrapolation of the data suggests that most patients under 60 years of age will gain about 10 years of extra life.

Complications

Short term

- Delayed function: occurs in up to 30% when obstruction and vascular problems must be excluded. A biopsy is usually performed if there is no recovery by 1 week to look for rejection.

- Technical problems: ureteric necrosis or stenosis usually relate to ischaemia and occur in 3–5%. Renal arterial and venous thrombosis often relate to technical problems.
- Acute rejection: occurs in about 30%. Diagnosed on renal biopsy (Fig. 69). First-line treatment is intravenous methylprednisolone. Second-line treatment involves anti-T-cell agents (e.g. antithymocyte globulin or OKT3).
- Infection: cytomegalovirus (CMV) is the most common problem and produces substantial morbidity and some mortality. Fungal pathogens, such as PCP, aspergillosis and systemic candidiasis, are rare but have a high case fatality rate (Fig. 70).

Long term

- Cardiovascular disease: very common (at least 30%). Risk factors include diabetes, calcific arterial disease and hypertension. Calineurin inhibitors and corticosteroids are both associated with worsening hypertension and hyperlipidaemia.
- Chronic graft dysfunction: although 1-year graft survival has improved, long-term attrition remains a major problem. Immunological and non-immunological mechanisms are probably involved. Average graft survival is 10–12 years.
- Diabetes: this develops in up to 10% of patients. Factors include steroids and calcineurin inhibitors (especially tacrolimus).
- Malignancy: skin cancers are very common. Post-transplantation lymphoproliferative disorder (PTLD) is a particular concern, and clearly associated with the intensity of immunosuppression. Most commonly of B-cell origin and often related to Epstein–Barr virus (EBV). Incidence of most other solid tumours is also significantly increased.

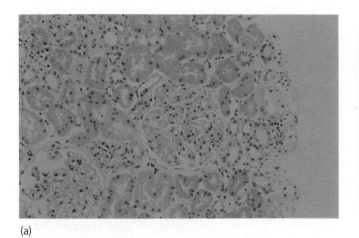

(a)

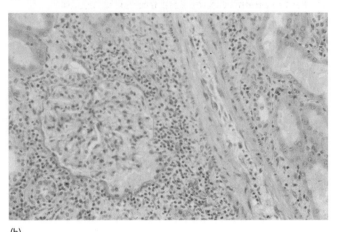

(b)

Fig. 69 Renal transplant biopsy: (a) normal kidney; (b) intense mononuclear cellular infiltrate together with arteritis consistent with acute severe rejection.

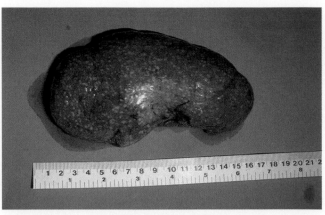

(a)

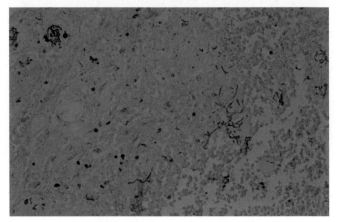

(b)

Fig. 70 Transplant nephrectomy specimen from a patient who died of systemic candidiasis 3 months after transplantation. (a) Macroscopic view shows multiple small abscesses studded over the surface of the kidney. (b) Microscopy reveals filamentous fungal hyphae morphologically consistent with *Candida* species. Blood cultures grew *Candida albicans*.

Important information for patients

The information needs to be balanced and detailed. In the case of living donors, there is the additional responsibility of a healthy individual being subjected to an operation. An approved tissue typing tester must confirm that there is no reason to dispute the claimed relationship between a potential lining related donor and recipient. The Unrelated Living Transplant Regulatory Authority (ULTRA) must sanction all transplants between unrelated individuals. A multi-disciplinary approach is required involving transplant surgeons, renal physicians, transplant coordinators and specialist nursing staff. See *Immunology and immunosuppression*, Section 8.

1 Morris PJ. *Kidney Transplantation: Principles and practice*, 4th edn. Philadelphia: WB Saunders, 1994.
2 Suthanthiran M, Strom TB. Renal transplantation. *N Engl J Med* 1994; 331: 365–376.
3 Wolfe RA, Ashby VB, Milford EL *et al.* Comparison of mortality in all patients on dialysis, patients on dialysis awaiting transplantation, and recipients of a first cadaveric transplant. *N Engl J Med* 1999; 341: 1725.

2.3 Glomerular diseases

Although many different diseases act on the glomeruli, the effects of glomerular damage are limited and include the following:

• Reduced glomerular filtration
• Proteinuria and haematuria
• Hypertension
• Sodium retention causing oedema.

Glomerular disease can seem confusing, partly because it can be classified according to the clinical syndrome, the histopathological appearance or the underlying disease. Glomerular disease can affect one or more of these components:

• Glomerular basement membrane
• Glomerular cells
• Intraglomerular vessels
• Mesangium.

Further:
- In proliferative disease, there is proliferation of cells within the glomerulus. In severe cases, proliferation of cells, especially macrophages within Bowman's capsule, causes an appearance known as a crescent.
- In mesangial disease, there is excess production of mesangial matrix.
- In membranous disease, the glomerular basement membrane is damaged and thickened.
- Membranoproliferative disease causes both thickening of the glomerular basement membrane and cellular proliferation, usually of mesangial cells.

- Focal disease affects only some glomeruli
- Diffuse disease affects all the glomeruli
- Segmental disease affects only part of the glomerulus
- Global disease affects the whole glomerulus.

O'Callaghan CA, Brenner BM. *The Kidney at a Glance.* Oxford: Blackwell Science, 2000.

2.3.1 PRIMARY GLOMERULAR DISEASE

Minimal change nephropathy

Aetiology/pathophysiology/pathology

The cause is unknown but is associated with atopy.
- Light microscopy and immunofluorescence are normal
- Electron microscopy shows glomerular epithelial podocyte foot process fusion (Fig. 3).

Epidemiology

This constitutes 80% of childhood nephrotic syndrome, 25% of adult nephrotic syndrome with an incidence of 2 per 100 000. Peak ages 2–7 years, but all ages can be affected.

Clinical presentation

- Nephrotic syndrome: often follows upper respiratory tract infection.

Physical signs

- Oedema
- Often facial swelling in children.

Investigations

- Urinalysis: protein—nephrotic range on 24-h collection
- Plasma: hypoalbuminaemia, hyperlipidaemia

- Renal biopsy: children are often treated with a trial of steroids without a biopsy.

Differential diagnosis

The differential diagnosis is from other causes of the nephrotic syndrome especially FSGS and membranous nephropathy, amyloidosis, diabetic nephropathy, lupus and, rarely, congenital nephrotic syndrome.

Treatment

- Steroids: if frequent relapses or poor response, then cyclophosphamide or cyclosporin can be useful
- Diuretics for oedema
- Lipid-lowering drugs (usually HMG-CoA reductase inhibitors), if prolonged nephrotic syndrome with hyperlipidaemia
- Penicillin prophylaxis may be given for streptococcal infection.

Complications

Complications are those of the nephrotic syndrome (see Section 2.1.4, pp. 58–61).

Prognosis

Ninety-eight per cent of children and 94% of adults respond to steroids, 10–20% of these relapse several times, of whom 40–50% relapse frequently.

Disease associations

- Lymphoma
- NSAID use.

Focal segmental glomerulosclerosis

Aetiology/pathophysiology/pathology

This is of unknown aetiology. Minimal change nephropathy and FSGS share similarities and may be different points on the spectrum of a disease process. Damage to the glomerular filtration barrier causes protein leak and nephrotic syndrome.
- Light microscopy: focal and segmental glomerular sclerosis
- Immunofluorescence: IgM and C3 in scars
- Electron microscopy: glomerular epithelial podocyte foot process fusion.

Epidemiology

This accounts for 15% of adult nephrotic syndrome.

73

Clinical presentation

Clinical presentations may include:
- Proteinuria
- Nephrotic syndrome
- Hypertension
- Chronic renal impairment.

Physical signs

- Hypertension
- Oedema if nephrotic.

Investigations

- Urinalysis: protein ± blood
- Plasma: hypoalbuminaemia and renal impairment
- Renal biopsy.

Differential diagnosis

The differential diagnosis is from other causes of nephrotic syndrome or renal impairment (if present).

Treatment

- Steroids are beneficial in some cases
- Cyclosporin or cyclophosphamide may be beneficial
- Symptomatic treatment: diuretics, ACE inhibitors to control blood pressure and reduce proteinuria, lipid-lowering agents.

Complications

Complications are those of the nephrotic syndrome and chronic renal impairment (see Section 2.1.2, pp. 50–56). Often recurs in transplanted kidneys.

Prognosis

- 40–60% develop end-stage renal disease within 10 years of diagnosis. Up to 40% of both adults and children remit in response to steroids: those who do respond have a better prognosis for renal survival.

Disease associations

FSGS occurs at increased frequency in black, HIV-infected, intravenous drug users. Also associated with obesity.

Membranous nephropathy

Aetiology/pathophysiology/pathology

The aetiology is unknown. Damage to the glomerular filtration barrier causes protein leak and nephrotic syndrome.
- Light microscopy: thickening of the glomerular basement membrane
- Immunofluorescence: immunoglobulin and complement deposition
- Electron microscopy: subepithelial membrane deposits.

Epidemiology

This is the most common cause of adult nephrotic syndrome in the UK. The peak age is 30–50 years.

Clinical presentation

Clinical presentations may include:
- Nephrotic syndrome
- Chronic renal impairment
- Asymptomatic proteinuria
- Hypertension.

Physical signs

- Oedema if nephrotic
- Hypertension.

Investigations

- Urinalysis: protein ± blood
- Plasma: hypoalbuminaemia, renal impairment
- Renal biopsy.

Differential diagnosis

The differential diagnosis is from other causes of nephrotic syndrome or renal impairment (if present). Exclude systemic lupus erythematosus.

Treatment

- Steroids and chlorambucil (the Ponticelli regimen) can slow the loss of renal function; cyclophosphamide has been used instead of chlorambucil
- Symptomatic treatment: diuretics, ACE inhibitors to control blood pressure, lipid-lowering agents.

Complications

Complications are those of the nephrotic syndrome, chronic renal impairment and hyperlipidaemia if present.

Prognosis

Twenty to thirty per cent remit spontaneously. Forty per cent have a partial remission or remain stable; around 30% develop progressive renal failure.

Disease associations

- Hepatitis B
- Malignancy
- SLE
- Drugs (gold and penicillamine, mercury).

IgA nephropathy

Aetiology/pathophysiology/pathology

This is of unknown aetiology—associated with abnormal glycosylation of the hinge region of bone marrow-derived IgA. Renal IgA deposition may trigger complement-mediated damage.
- Light microscopy: mesangial matrix expansion and mesangial cell proliferation (Fig. 112)
- Immunofluorescence: IgA deposits in mesangium (Fig. 112).

Epidemiology

This is relatively common—prevalence of 2 per 10 000. Postmortem studies revealed similar changes in 2–5%. Peak in second and third decades. M : F = 3.6 : 1.

Clinical presentation

There may be macroscopic haematuria at the same time as or 1–2 days after a sore throat (synpharyngitic); there is also asymptomatic microscopic haematuria, hypertension and renal impairment, less commonly nephrotic syndrome and rarely acute nephritis.

Physical signs

- Hypertension.

Investigations

- Urinalysis: blood, protein
- Plasma: renal impairment, serum IgA raised in 50% of cases
- Renal biopsy.

Differential diagnosis

The differential diagnosis can be other forms of glomerulonephritis.

Treatment

The role of treatment is unclear. Benefit is claimed for ACE inhibitors, fish oils and steroids.
- Steroids may be given if nephrotic
- Aggressive disease with crescent formation may be treated with steroids and cyclophosphamide
- Symptomatic treatment: diuretics, hypertension (ACE inhibitors), lipid-lowering agents.

Complications

Complications are those of the nephrotic syndrome or chronic renal impairment (if present).

Prognosis

Highly variable from remission to rapid progression to end-stage renal disease: 15% develop end-stage renal disease by 10 years; 20–30% develop it by 20 years.

Disease associations

- Liver disease: alcoholic and viral hepatitis
- HIV-associated IgA nephropathy
- Coeliac disease.

Mesangiocapillary glomerulonephritis (or membranoproliferative glomerulonephritis)

Aetiology/pathophysiology/pathology

This is of unknown aetiology, although, if cryoglobulinaemia is present, hepatitis C is often the underlying cause. Subclassified into types I and II:
- Light microscopy: types I and II—mesangial expansion and mesangial cell proliferation, thickening of the glomerular basement membrane
- Immunofluorescence: type I—immunoglobulins and complement; type II—some C3
- Electron microscopy: type I—subendothelial deposits; type II—intramembranous deposits, subepithelial deposits.

Epidemiology

This is declining in developed countries; 80% of cases are of type I. It accounts for 10–20% of biopsies performed for presumed primary glomerulonephritis.

Clinical presentation

Presentation varies from asymptomatic haematuria or proteinuria to acute nephritis or severe nephrotic syndrome.

Physical signs

- Hypertension
- Oedema.

Investigations

- Urinalysis: blood, protein
- Plasma: renal impairment, hypoalbuminaemia; low complement levels, especially C3. In type II disease there may be antibodies to the C3 convertase C3bBb, resulting in complement activation
- Renal biopsy.

Differential diagnosis

The differential diagnosis is from other causes of chronic renal impairment and of nephrotic syndrome (if present). Both post-infectious glomerulonephritis and systemic lupus erythematosus (SLE) can cause renal disease and hypocomplementaemia.

Treatment

Treat any underlying cause:
- Although steroids and cytotoxic agents have been used, their benefit has not been proved in adults
- Symptomatic treatment: diuretics, ACE inhibitors to control blood pressure, lipid-lowering agents.

Complications

Complications are those of the nephrotic syndrome or chronic renal impairment (if present). There is a high recurrence rate in renal transplantation.

Prognosis

Fifty per cent develop end-stage renal disease by 10 years; 90% develop it by 20 years.

Disease associations

- Infection, especially with hepatitis B and C viruses
- Autoimmune disease, especially SLE
- Complement deficiency: partial lipodystrophy is associated with type II disease
- Hypogammaglobulinaemia.

Diffuse proliferative glomerulonephritis (or acute endocapillary glomerulonephritis)

Aetiology/pathophysiology/pathology

This may be idiopathic or secondary to infection (typically poststreptococcal).
- Light microscopy: endothelial and mesangial cell proliferation, glomerular infiltration with neutrophils and monocytes
- Immunofluorescence: complement and immunoglobulins
- Electron microscopy: subepithelial deposits.

Epidemiology

This is declining in developing countries. Peak age 2–12 years, M : F = 2 : 1. It accounts for 10% of glomerular disease in developed countires, and is the most common histological presentation of intrinsic renal disease in developing countries.

Clinical presentation

Presentation is typically 1–2 weeks after a streptococcal throat infection or 3–6 weeks after a streptococcal skin infection. It varies from asymptomatic microscopic haematuria to acute nephritic syndrome with frank haematuria, oedema, hypertension and oliguria.

Physical signs

- Hypertension
- Oedema
- Signs of preceding infection.

Investigations

- Urinalysis: blood (all cases), sometimes protein, often red blood cell casts
- Plasma: impaired renal function; serological evidence of infection such as raised antistreptolysin O titres. Low complement levels, especially C3.

Differential diagnosis

- Mesangiocapillary glomerulonephritis
- SLE.

Treatment

- Ensure that infection is eradicated (antibiotics, surgery)
- Symptomatic treatment: diuretics, hypertension (ACE inhibitors), lipid-lowering agents.

Complications

Complications are those of the ongoing infection, uncontrolled oedema or hypertension.

Prognosis

- Good: only 0.1–1% have progressive renal impairment.

Antiglomerular basement membrane disease (or Goodpasture's disease)

Aetiology/pathophysiology/pathology

Autoantibodies to the basement membrane in glomeruli and alveoli cause renal and pulmonary damage. The antigen is usually part of the non-collagenous domain of the α_3 component of type IV collagen.
- Light microscopy: focal segmental proliferative glomerulonephritis, often with necrosis and crescents
- Immunofluorescence: antibody deposition (usually IgG) along the glomerular basement membrane.

Epidemiology

This is rare: 0.5–1 per million. It occurs mainly in white patients; M >F.

Clinical presentation

The presentation is with lung haemorrhage in 50–70% of patients causing cough, haemoptysis or shortness of breath. Renal involvement is initially asymptomatic, but can cause loin pain, frank haematuria, oliguria and acute renal failure.

Physical signs

- Lung signs resemble pulmonary oedema or infection.

Investigations

- Urinalysis: blood and protein, red cell casts
- Plasma: renal impairment, antiglomerular basement membrane (GBM) antibodies
- Chest radiography: diffuse pulmonary haemorrhage may resemble pulmonary oedema or infection
- Lung function: gas transfer (KCO) is raised by the absorption of carbon monoxide by the blood in the alveoli if haemorrhage has occured recently
- Renal biopsy.

Differential diagnosis

- Systemic vasculitis

- Another glomerulonephritis with pulmonary oedema or infection.

Treatment

If the patient's kidneys have not failed completely:
- Plasma exchange is used to remove the pathogenic antibody
- Immunosuppression with steroids and cyclophosphamide is used to inhibit further antibody production and reduce inflammatory damage. Azathioprine may be substituted for cyclophosphamide in the later stages of treatment
- If the patient requires dialysis at presentation them most nephrologists would not give immunosuppression.

Complications

- Respiratory failure; secondary pulmonary infection; treatment toxicity.

Prognosis

Untreated, most patients die. Patients who require dialysis before treatment is started do not usually recover renal function and morbidity from immunosuppression is high (if given). If plasma creatinine is <600 µmol/L before treatment, 80–90% of patients recover independent renal function.

Disease associations

There is a strong association with HLA-DR15 and weaker association with HLA-DR4. Pulmonary haemorrhage is more common if the patient is a smoker, has pulmonary infection or oedema, or there is exposure to other inhaled toxins.

Crescentic glomerulonephritis (or rapidly progressive glomerulonephritis, focal necrotizing glomerulonephritis or renal microscopic polyangiitis)

Aetiology/pathophysiology/pathology

The aetiology varies.
- Light microscopy: shows a proliferative glomerulonephritis with fibrinoid necrosis often with crescents (inflammatory cells in Bowman's capsule) and may show small vessel vasculitis
- Immunofluorescence: see below.
  This condition is subclassified as follows:
- Antiglomerular basement membrane disease
- Renal microscopic vasculitis: immunofluorescence—

scant or absent immunoglobulins. Serum antineutrophil cytoplasmic antibody (ANCA) usually positive (see Sections 1.12, pp. 36–38 and 2.7.6, p. 97). There may or may not be extrarenal manifestations

• Complicating a pre-existing glomerulonephritis, a systemic disorder or an infection: immunofluorescence—often immunoglobulin deposition (associations include lupus, Henoch–Schönlein purpura, IgA nephropathy, mesangiocapillary glomerulonephritis and post-infectious glomerulonephritis).

Epidemiology

This accounts for 2–5% of renal biopsies; M : F = 2 : 1.

Clinical presentation

Renal disease is often asymptomatic but can result in oliguria and acute renal failure. Manifestations of associated or underlying systemic diseases may be present. There may be systemic symptoms such as fever, weight loss and general malaise.

Physical signs

Manifestations of systemic disease may be present, such as rashes or joint lesions.

Investigations

• Urinalysis: blood, protein and red blood cell casts
• Plasma: renal impairment; raised inflammatory markers such as CRP, ESR, white cell count and platelet count; positive serological tests for associated systemic diseases, especially ANCA or anti-GBM antibody
• Renal biopsy.

Differential diagnosis

• Other forms of acute glomerulonephritis.
• Other causes of acute renal failure.

Treatment

• Immunosuppression with prednisolone and cyclophosphamide, azathioprine may be substituted for cyclophosphamide after 3 months
• Plasma exchange is usually reserved for anti-GBM antibody disease.

Complications

Complications are those of immunosuppression and acute renal failure.

Prognosis

Less than 25% escape dialysis but, with treatment, the 5-year survival rate off dialysis is 60–80%.

Disease associations

See Aetiology above.

Minimal change nephropathy

Mak SK, Short CD, Mallick NP. Long-term outcome of adult-onset minimal-change nephropathy. *Nephrol Dial Transplant* 1996; 11: 2192–2201.

Fujimoto S, Yamamoto Y, Hisanaga S, Morita S, Eto T, Tanaka K. Minimal change nephrotic syndrome in adults: response to corticosteroid therapy and frequency of relapse. *Am J Kidney Dis* 1991; 17: 687–692.

Focal segmental glomerulosclerosis

Banfi G, Moriggi M, Sabadini E, Fellin G, D'Amico G, Ponticelli C. The impact of prolonged immunosuppression on the outcome of idiopathic focal-segmental glomerulosclerosis. *Clin Nephrol* 1991; 36: 53.

Cattran DC, Appel GB, Hebert LA *et al.* A randomized trial of cyclosporin in patients with steroid-resistant focal segmental glomerulosclerosis. *Kidney Int* 1999; 56: 2220–2226.

Membranous nephropathy

Ponticelli C, Zucchelli P, Passerini P, Cesana B. Methylprednisolone plus chlorambucil as compared with methylprednisolone alone for the treatment of idiopathic membranous nephropathy. *N Engl J Med* 1992; 327: 599–603.

Ponticelli C, Zucchelli P, Passerini P *et al.* A randomized trial of methylprednisolone and chlorambucil in idiopathic membranous nephropathy. *N Engl J Med* 1989; 320: 8–13.

Schieppati A, Mosconi L, Perna A *et al.* Prognosis of untreated patients with idiopathic membranous nephropathy. *N Engl J Med* 1993; 329: 85–89.

IgA nephropathy

Donadio JV, Bergstralh EJ, Offord KP, Spencer DC, Holley KE. A controlled trial of fish oil in IgA nephropathy. Mayo Nephrology Collaborative Group. *N Engl J Med* 1994; 331: 1194–1199.

Harper L, Savage CO. Treatment of IgA nephropathy. *Lancet* 1999; 353: 860–862.

Mesangiocapillary glomerulonephritis

Zamurovic C, Churg J. Idiopathic and secondary mesangiocapillary glomerulonephritis. *Nephron* 1984; 38: 145–153.

Cameron JS, Turner DR, Heaton J *et al.* Idiopathic mesangiocapillary glomerulonephritis. Comparison of types I and II in children and adults and long-term prognosis. *Am J Med* 1983; 74: 175–192.

Diffuse proliferative glomerulonephritis

Montseny JJ, Meyrier A, Kleinknecht D, Callard P. The current spectrum of infections glomerulonephritis. Experience with 76 patients and review of the literature. *Medicine (Baltimore)* 1995; 74: 63–73.

Antiglomerular basement membrane disease

Turner AN, Rees AJ. Goodpasture's disease and Alport's syndromes. *Annu Rev Med* 1996; 47: 377–386.

Crescentic glomerulonephritis

Jindal KK. Management of idiopathic crescentic and diffuse proliferative glomerulonephritis: evidence-based recommendations. *Kidney Int* 1999; suppl 70: S33–40.

Angangco R, Thiru S, Zsnault VL, Short AK, Lockwood CM, Oliveira DB. Does truly idiopathic crescentic glomerulonephritis exist? *Nephrol Dial Transplant* 1994; 9: 630–636.

2.3.2 SECONDARY GLOMERULAR DISEASE

Glomerular disease can be secondary to many conditions, including those discussed in Section 2.7, pp. 92–102. Malignancy and infection-associated glomerular disease are considered here.

Aetiology/pathophysiology/pathology

Malignancy-associated glomerulonephritis

The mechanism is unclear, but renal disease may improve with treatment of the malignancy. Most patterns of glomerulonephritis can occur.

Infection-related glomerulonephritis

The mechanism is usually unclear; pathogen antigens can trigger an aberrant immune response causing renal damage. Most patterns of glomerulonephritis can occur.

Epidemiology

Malignancy-associated glomerulonephritis

Of patients with malignancy, 15–58% have urinary abnormalities. Up to 17% of patients with solid tumours have histologically evident glomerular changes. Membranous nephropathy is the most common histological type.

Infection-related glomerulonephritis

Important problems can be associated with viral infection (hepatitis C, hepatitis B, HIV), bacterial infection (streptococcal, endocarditis) and other infections (malaria, syphilis).

Clinical presentation and physical signs

Malignancy-associated glomerulonephritis

This varies from asymptomatic urinary abnormality to nephrotic syndrome or acute renal failure. Physical signs depend on the tumour and the renal pathology.

Infection-related glomerulonephritis

This is highly variable, depending on the infection and its associated renal disease.

Investigations

These are as for other glomerular disease (see Section 2.3.1, pp. 73–78). Investigations will also be directed towards the malignancy or infection.

Differential diagnosis

Malignancy-associated glomerulonephritis

The differential diagnosis is from primary glomerulonephritis and other tumour-related causes of renal dysfunction, including obstruction, invasion of the renal tract, renal vein thrombosis, urate nephropathy, hypercalcaemia and drug toxicity.

Infection-related glomerulonephritis

Differential diagnosis is from unrelated primary glomerulonephritis. With chronic infection, AA amyloidosis can occur. In treated infections, consider drug toxicity.

Treatment

• Treat the malignancy in malignancy-associated glomerulonephritis
• Eradicate, where possible, the infection in infection-related glomerulonephritis.

Complications

Malignancy-associated glomerulonephritis

The complications are those of the malignancy and its therapy, as well as of the nephrotic syndrome, hypertension or renal impairment if present.

Infection-related glomerulonephritis

The complications are those of the underlying infection, also the nephrotic syndrome, hypertension and renal impairment if present.

Prognosis

This depends on the infection or malignancy. Generally, renal involvement is associated with a worsened prognosis for the malignancy.

Disease associations

Infection-related glomerulonephritis

- Hepatitis B: membranous nephropathy, mesangiocapillary glomerulonephritis (type I), IgA nephropathy
- Hepatitis C: mesangiocapillary glomerulonephritis (type I), mixed essential cryoglobulinaemia type II
- HIV: focal segmental glomerulosclerosis
- EBV: microscopic haematuria and proteinuria
- Streptococcal infection: poststreptococcal (diffuse proliferative) glomerulonephritis
- Staphylococcal infection (endocarditis, shunt infections, general sepsis): diffuse proliferative glomerulonephritis or focal segmental proliferative glomerulonephritis, or type I mesangiocapillary glomerulonephritis
- Salmonella infections: mesangiocapillary glomerulonephritis or IgA nephropathy
- Tuberculosis: amyloidosis
- Leprosy: amyloidosis or diffuse proliferative glomerulonephritis or mesangiocapillary glomerulonephritis
- Malaria, syphilis: membranous nephropathy
- *Escherichia coli* and other enteric infections can cause haemolytic uraemic syndrome (see Section 2.7.3, p. 94)
- Leptospirosis causes an acute tubulointerstitial nephritis.

Bennet WM. Paraneoplastic glomerulopathies. *Semin Nephrol* 1993; 13: 258–272.

Daghestani L, Pomeroy C. Renal manifestations of hepatitis C infection. *Am J Med* 1999; 106: 347–354.

Humphreys MH. Human immunodeficiency virus associated glomerulosclerosis. *Kidney Int* 1995; 48: 311–320.

2.4 Tubulointerstitial diseases

2.4.1 ACUTE TUBULAR NECROSIS

Pathophysiology

Most cases result from hypoperfusion injury following renal ischaemia (Fig. 71). After an ischaemic insult there is intense afferent arteriolar vasoconstriction, mediated by vasoconstrictors (e.g. endothelin), and loss of intrinsic vasodilators (e.g. nitric oxide and prostacyclin [PGI_2]). The cells of the proximal tubule are particularly susceptible to damage: cell necrosis mediated by calcium and oxygen free radicals results in cell shedding from the tubular basement membrane, with formation of casts that can block urine flow (Figs 72 and 73). The tubular cells can regenerate provided that the tubular basement membrane remains intact.

Epidemiology

Acute renal failure (ARF) requiring dialysis has an overall annual incidence of about 70 cases/million and over 50% of these are caused by ATN. Elderly people are at much higher risk.

Clinical presentation

Acute renal failure, which may be non-oliguric. ATN is often part of the multi-organ failure (MOF) syndrome.

Investigations

- Urine may show protein trace/+ and/or blood trace/+, but heavy proteinuria, heavy haematuria and cellular casts are not a feature
- Ultrasonography shows normal-size unobstructed kidneys
- Renal biopsy is not usually necessary, but if performed shows tubular necrosis, sometimes with evidence of regeneration.

Treatment

- The first priority is treatment of life-threatening complications (see Section 1.6, pp. 16–19)
- Supportive: maintain circulation and oxygenation, and avoid nephrotoxic drugs.

  Some nephrologists give a trial of high-dose furosemide (frusemide) (500 mg over 4 hours IV) with dopamine (2.5 μg 1 kg IV), but there is no proof of efficacy.
- Dialysis should be commenced at an early stage; patients with MOF need to be managed on the ICU
- The precipitating condition must be treated vigorously.

Prognosis

Approximately 60% of all patients who require renal replacement therapy for ARF will survive. Of the survivors, 60% will regain full renal function, but 30% have residual CRF and 10% end-stage renal failure.

Kalra PA. Acute renal failure. In: *Renal Disease: Prevention and Treatment* (Raman GV, Golper TA, eds). London: Chapman & Hall, 1998: 293–324.

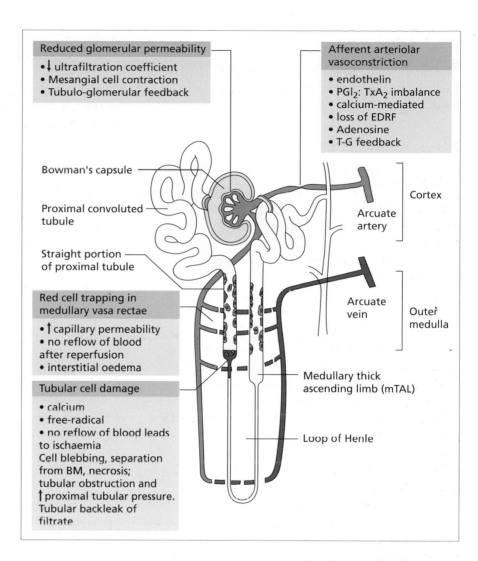

Reduced glomerular permeability

- $\downarrow$ ultrafiltration coefficient
- Mesangial cell contraction
- Tubulo-glomerular feedback

Afferent arteriolar vasoconstriction

- endothelin
- PGI_2: TxA_2 imbalance
- calcium-mediated
- loss of EDRF
- Adenosine
- T-G feedback

Bowman's capsule

Proximal convoluted tubule

Straight portion of proximal tubule

Red cell trapping in medullary vasa rectae

- $\uparrow$ capillary permeability
- no reflow of blood after reperfusion
- interstitial oedema

Tubular cell damage

- calcium
- free-radical
- no reflow of blood leads to ischaemia

Cell blebbing, separation from BM, necrosis; tubular obstruction and $\uparrow$ proximal tubular pressure. Tubular backleak of filtrate

Cortex

Arcuate artery

Arcuate vein

Outer medulla

Medullary thick ascending limb (mTAL)

Loop of Henle

Fig. 71 Schema summarizing the pathophysiology of ischaemic ARF.

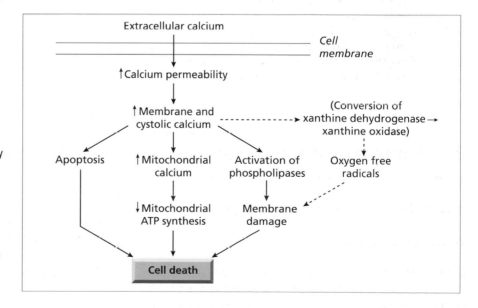

Extracellular calcium

Cell membrane

$\uparrow$ Calcium permeability

$\uparrow$ Membrane and cystolic calcium

(Conversion of xanthine dehydrogenase → xanthine oxidase)

Apoptosis

$\uparrow$ Mitochondrial calcium

Activation of phospholipases

Oxygen free radicals

$\downarrow$ Mitochondrial ATP synthesis

Membrane damage

Cell death

Fig. 72 Role of calcium in the pathophysiology of ATN. The intracellular calcium concentration is normally much lower than that of the extracellular compartment. As a result of ischaemia, cellular membrane integrity is reduced, calcium enters the cell and overloads the intrinsic buffering systems (the mitochondria). Hence, the energy charge of the cell drops, allowing sodium and water influx with accompanying cell swelling and lysis.

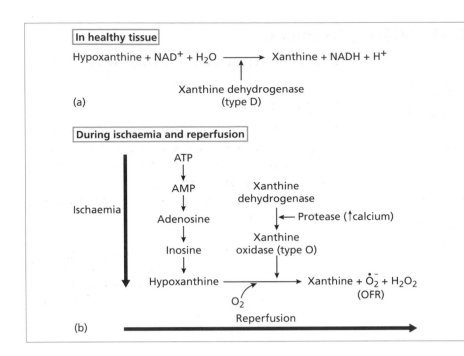

(a) **In healthy tissue**

$$Hypoxanthine + NAD^+ + H_2O \longrightarrow Xanthine + NADH + H^+$$

Xanthine dehydrogenase
(type D)

(b) **During ischaemia and reperfusion**

Ischaemia

ATP ↓ AMP ↓ Adenosine ↓ Inosine ↓ Hypoxanthine

Xanthine dehydrogenase ← Protease (↑calcium)
Xanthine oxidase (type O)

$$Hypoxanthine \longrightarrow Xanthine + \dot{O}_2^- + H_2O_2$$
(OFR)

O_2^-

Reperfusion

Fig. 73 The generation of oxygen free radicals (OFRs) in ischaemia/reperfusion. (a) Hypoxanthine (purine breakdown product) metabolism in normal conditions. (b) During ischaemia, ATP is degraded rapidly to hypoxanthine, which increases by many-fold. A calcium-mediated conversion favours formation of the xanthine oxidase (type O) enzyme over xanthine dehydrogenase (type D), and XO cannot interact with NAD⁺. However, in the presence of molecular oxygen, which returns to the tissue during reperfusion, the formation of the OFRs, superoxide and peroxide is catalysed. The OFRs attack cellular membranes, leading to increased permeability.

2.4.2 ACUTE INTERSTITIAL NEPHRITIS

Aetiology

Some cases are idiopathic, but a recognized precipitating cause (most often drugs, particularly antibiotics or NSAIDs) can be found in most patients.

Causes of acute interstitial nephritis

- Idiopathic
- Drugs, e.g. NSAIDs (most common cause), penicillin, rifampicin, allopurinol, cephalosporins, sulphonamides, furosemide (frusemide), thiazide diuretics, cimetidine, amphotericin
- Infections: viral (e.g. Hanta virus), bacterial (e.g. leptospirosis), mycobacterial.

Clinical presentation

This is usually with mild renal impairment and hypertension or, in more severe cases, ARF, which is often non-oliguric [1]. Systemic manifestations may include fever, arthralgia and skin rash.

Investigations

- Urinalysis may be unremarkable (e.g. minor proteinuria); urinary eosinophils may be present
- Differential FBC may show an eosinophilia and serum IgE can be raised
- Renal biopsy typically shows oedema of the interstitium with infiltration of plasma cells, lymphocytes and eosinophils (Fig. 74).

Treatment

Treatment involves cessation of the precipitating cause (e.g. drugs), and moderate-dose oral steroids in selected cases.

Prognosis

Most patients make a complete renal recovery.

Droz D, Kleinknecht D. Acute interstitial nephritis. In: Davison AM, Cameron JS, Grünfeld J-P, Kerr DNS, Ritz E, Winearis CG (eds) *Oxford Textbook of Clinical Nephrology* (2nd edn). Oxford: Oxford University Press, 1998: 1634–1648.

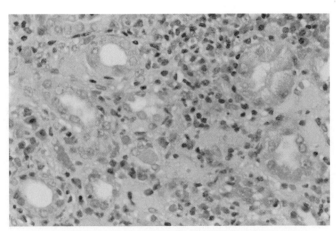

Fig. 74 Histological appearance of acute interstitial nephritis. There is a diffuse inflammatory infiltrate with plasma cells and lymphocytes; tubular architecture is well preserved (H&E, ×200).

2.4.3 CHRONIC INTERSTITIAL NEPHRITIS

Aetiology

Diverse systemic or renal conditions and drugs can result in chronic inflammation within the tubulointerstitium.

> **Causes of chronic interstitial nephritis**
>
> • Immunological diseases: SLE, Sjögren's syndrome, rheumatoid arthritis, systemic sclerosis
> • Granulomatous disease: Wegener's granulomatosis, tuberculosis (TB), sarcoidosis
> • Drugs: cyclosporin A, cisplatin, lithium, iron, analgesics
> • Haematological disorders: myeloma, light-chain nephropathy, sickle cell disease
> • Chronic infections: TB
> • Heavy metals: lead, cadmium
> • Hereditary disorders: nephronophthisis, Alport's syndrome
> • Metabolic disorders: hypercalcaemia, hypokalaemia, hyperuricaemia
> • Endemic disease: Balkan nephropathy
> • Other: irradiation, chronic transplant rejection.

Clinical presentation

Patients present with CRF or end-stage renal failure. Some patients may also manifest renal tubular acidosis (usually type 1) (see Section 2.4.4), nephrogenic diabetes insipidus or salt-wasting states.

Investigations

Renal biopsy shows a chronic inflammatory infiltrate within the interstitium, often with extensive scarring and tubular loss (Fig. 75); the latter indicates irreversible renal damage.

Other histological features may be specific to the underlying disorder (see Section 2.7, pp. 92–102):
• Tubular casts with myeloma or light-chain nephropathy
• Granulomas in TB or sarcoidosis.

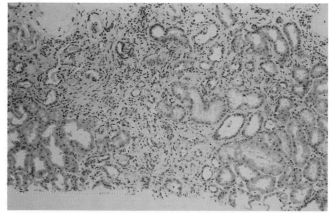

Fig. 75 Histological appearance of chronic interstitial nephritis. Alongside the inflammatory infiltrate, there is evidence of chronic tubulointerstitial damage, with scarring and tubular atrophy (H&E, ×80).

Treatment

Treat the underlying condition. Withdraw drug/toxin.

Prognosis

This depends on the cause and the severity of damage at the time of diagnosis. If the cause can be treated (e.g. connective tissue disorder) or removed (e.g. drugs), then progression of the CRF may be prevented [1]. However, extensive tubulointerstitial fibrosis usually predicts a progressive decline to end-stage renal failure.

1 Tse Wy, Adu D. Non-steroidal anti-inflammatory drugs and the kidney. In: Davison AM, Cameron JS, Grünfeld J-P, Kerr DNS, Ritz E, Winearls CG (eds) *Oxford Textbook of Clinical Nephrology* (2nd edn). Oxford: Oxford University Press, 1998: 1147–1156.

2.4.4 SPECIFIC TUBULOINTERSTITIAL DISORDERS

Balkan nephropathy

Aetiology

This was initially thought to be a toxic nephropathy (e.g. trace metals in water) or viral infection; recent evidence suggests chronic exposure to fungal toxin [1].

Epidemiology

This is a chronic interstitial renal disease endemic in villages along the tributaries of the river Danube (e.g. Romania, Bulgaria, Bosnia, Croatia).

Clinical presentation

Presentation is with CRF or end-stage renal failure.

Physical signs

Patients have coppery-yellow pigmentation of the palms and soles.

Investigations

Imaging reveals two small kidneys.

Treatment

As for CRF (see Section 2.1.2) and end-stage renal failure (see Section 2.1.3).

Complications

Urothelial malignancy is increased 200-fold.

Analgesic nephropathy

Aetiology

- Chronic analgesic usage (previously compound analgesics containing phenacetin, now NSAIDs) [2].

Epidemiology

Between 1950 and 1970, analgesic nephropathy was the most common cause of both ARF and CRF in parts of Europe and Australia. The condition is now in decline, especially since the withdrawal of phenacetin. Women are affected more often than men.

Clinical presentation

There is a history of chronic analgesic usage, e.g. for backache, pelvic inflammatory disease, headache. There may be loin pain associated with papillary necrosis. Presentation is often with CRF or end-stage renal failure.

Investigations

The classic radiological appearance of cup and spill calyces, resulting from papillary necrosis, with renal scarring is seen on IVU (Fig. 76). Renal biopsy is not of diagnostic value.

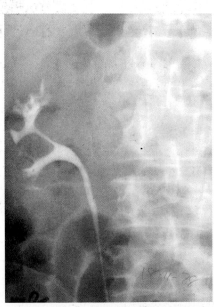

Fig. 76 IVU of papillary necrosis. There is clubbing of right upper polar calyces with typical 'cup and spill' deformities.

Treatment

As for CRF (see Section 2.1.2) and end-stage renal failure (see Section 2.1.3). Complete cessation of analgesic consumption. Prompt treatment of infection/obstruction.

Complications

The risk of urothelial malignancy is increased.

Renal tubular acidosis

Aetiology

- Distal or type 1 renal tubal acidosis (RTA) results from impaired urinary H^+ acidification
- Proximal or type 2 RTA is caused by a failure of bicarbonate reabsorption [3]
- Type 4 RTA (hyporeninaemic hypoaldosteronism) describes a metabolic acidosis that is associated with hyperkalaemia and mild renal impairment (GFR usually >30 mL/min).

Epidemiology

- Distal RTA is fairly common and can complicate many renal parenchymal disorders that predominantly affect the medullary regions
- Proximal RTA is uncommon.

The causes of different forms of RTA are shown in Table 22.

Table 22 Causes of renal tubular acidosis.

Type of RTA	Causes
Distal RTA	• Primary: genetic (dominant) or idiopathic • Secondary to autoimmune diseases: SLE, Sjögren's • Tubulointerstitial disease: Chronic pyelonephritis, transplant rejection, obstructive uropathy, chronic interstitial nephritis • Nephrocalcinosis: Medullary sponge kidney, hypercalcaemia • Drugs and toxins: lithium, amphotericin, toluene
Proximal RTA	• Occurring alone: idiopathic • With Fanconi syndrome: Wilson's disease, cystinosis, fructose intolerance, Sjögren's syndrome • Tubulointerstitial disease: interstitial nephritis, myeloma, amyloidosis • Drugs and toxins: outdated tetracyclines, streptozotocin, lead and mercury (and other heavy metals), acetazolamide, sulphonamides
Type IV RTA	• Diabetic nephropathy • Gouty nephropathy • Urinary tract obstruction • Drugs: NSAIDs or potassium-sparing diuretics

RTA, renal tubular acidosis.

Clinical presentation

Distal RTA can present with acidosis, hyperventilation and muscular weakness (due to hypokalaemia). Growth failure and rickets in children; osteomalacia in adults. Seventy per cent have nephrocalcinosis or urinary stones.

Proximal RTA can present with growth failure and rickets (children), osteomalacia (adults) and proximal myopathy. Polyuria and polydipsia can be seen.

Physical signs

The diagnosis of RTA depends on demonstrating that in the presence of normal or near-normal EFR the renal tubules cannot excrete acid normally. In many cases formal testing is not required, but determination of the minimum urinary pH after ingestion of a standardized dose of ammonium chloride can be used when needed: this should fall to less than pH5.5.
• Distal RTA: plasma bicarbonate tends to be very low (<12 mmol/L) and urinary pH is always >5.5. There may be severe hypokalaemia. Abdominal radiograph may show nephrocalcinosis/urinary stones.
• Proximal RTA: when plasma bicarbonate falls very low, urinary pH can fall to normal minimum (pH<5.3). Almost always associated with Fanconi syndrome (phosphaturia, glycosuria, aminociduria, uricosuria). Nephrocalcalcinosis and urinary stones are not seen. Hypokalaemia is common.

Treatment

• Distal RTA: the acutely acidotic patient is usually very hypokalaemic. Intravenous potassium must be given before bicarbonate. Chronic acidosis responds well to oral sodium bicarbonate (1–3 mmol/kg body wt/day)
• Proximal RTA: very large doses of oral sodium bicarbonate (3–20 mmol/kg body wt/day) are required, usually with potassium supplementation.

Complications

• Distal RTA: nephrocalcinosis (Fig. 77), calculi and growth failure
• Proximal RTA: rickets and osteomalacia (caused by phosphate wasting).

Reflux nephropathy (or chronic pyelonephritis)

Aetiology

Childhood vesicoureteric reflux (VUR) and infection cause renal scarring and nephropathy [4] (Fig. 78). There

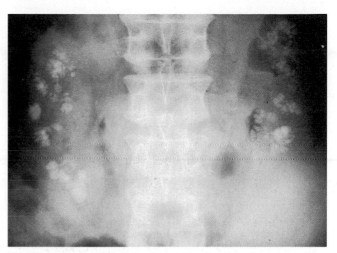

Fig. 77 Nephrocalcinosis. Plain abdominal radiograph of a patient with renal tubular acidosis. There is gross calcification within the outer medullary and cortical regions of the kidneys.

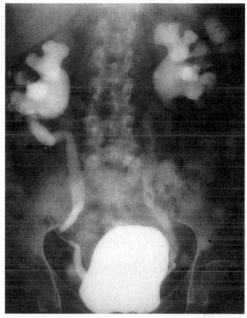

Fig. 78 Micturating cystogram showing severe reflux nephropathy (grade 3).

is a genetic predisposition, with children of parents with reflux nephropathy having a one in four chance of VUR.

Epidemiology

Vesicoureteric reflux is common during the first 5 years of life (when almost all scarring occurs), but diminishes with age. End-stage renal failure caused by reflux nephropathy accounts for about 15% of patients entering dialysis programmes.

Clinical presentation

In young children, VUR usually presents with a urinary tract infection [5]. Adults may present with hypertension, proteinuria or chronic renal impairment.

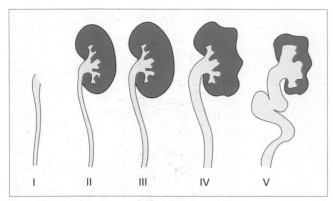

Fig. 79 Classification of vesicoureteric reflux. Grade I: ureter only. Grade II: up to pelvis and calyces, but with no dilatation. Grade III: mild-to-moderate dilatation, but with only minimal blunting of fornices. Grade IV: moderate dilatation, with obliteration of sharp angles of fornices. Grade V: gross dilatation and tortuosity of ureter and pelvicalcyceal system, and calyces severely clubbed.

The classic radiological appearance of cup and spill calyces, resulting from papillary necrosis, with renal scarring is seen on IVU (Fig. 77). Renal biopsy is not of diagnostic value.

Investigations

Diagnosis of VUR is by micturating cystography. Scarring can be demonstrated by ultrasonography or ^{99m}Tc-dimercaptosuccinic acid (DMSA) scintigraphy. Reflux can be graded from grade I (involving reflux into the ureter only) to grade V (gross dilatation and tortuosity of ureter, renal pelvis and calyces) (Fig. 79). It is recommended that offspring or siblings (if a child) of affected patients undergo screening.

Treatment

Renal scarring results from infection in young children. To try to prevent this, children with reflux are given antibiotic prophylaxis. Surgery for VUR is controversial; techniques include:
• Endoscopic injection of collagen behind the intravesical ureter
• Lengthening of the submucosal ureteric tunnel
• Ureteric reimplantation.
As with all forms of chronic, potentially progressive, renal disorders, hypertension must be properly controlled (see Section 2.1.2, pp. 50–56).

Complications

Prevention

Of children with a urinary tract infection (UTI), 15–60% will have some degree of VUR, and about 10% will have

evidence of reflux nephropathy. All children with a UTI should be investigated for VUR.

About 5% of women with symptomatic UTI will have reflux nephropathy.

1 Stefanovic V, Polenakovic MH. Balkan nephropathy. Kidney disease beyond the Balkans? *Am J Nephrol* 1991; 11: 1–11.
2 Nanra RS. Analgesic nephropathy in the 1990s—an Australian perspective. *Kidney Int* 1993; 42: S86–92.
3 Du Bose T, Alpern RJ. Renal tubular acidosis. In: *The Metabolic Basis of Inherited Disease*, 6th edn (Scriver CR, Beaudet AL, Sly WS, Valle D, eds). New York: McGraw-Hill, 1989.
4 Smellie JM, Edwards D, Hunter N, Normand ICS, Prescod N. Vesico-ureteric reflux and renal scarring. *Kidney Int* 1975; 8: S65–72.
5 Bailey RR. Vesicoureteric reflux and reflux nephropathy. In: Davison AM, Cameron JS, Grünfeld J-P, Kerr DNS, Ritz E, Winearls CG (eds) *Oxford Textbook of Clinical Nephrology* (2nd edn). Oxford: Oxford University Press, 1998: 2501–2521.

2.5 Diseases of renal vessels

2.5.1 RENOVASCULAR DISEASE

Aetiology

The overwhelming majority of patients have atheromatous renovascular disease (ARVD). Fibromuscular dysplasia is a rare cause of renal artery stenosis and hypertension in young patients.

Epidemiology

Atheromatous renovascular disease is associated with generalized vascular disease. It is present in 30% of patients undergoing coronary angiography and 59% with peripheral vascular disease, and it affects 34% of patients with congestive heart failure aged >70 years. As older patients are now readily admitted to dialysis programmes, ARVD is an increasing cause of end-stage renal failure (about 20%) [1].

Clinical presentation

Presentation is with hypertension (80% of all secondary hypertension, i.e. 4% of all cases of hypertension), CRF or end-stage renal failure, 'flash' pulmonary oedema and ACE inhibitor-related ARF (see Section 1.11, p. 34). Predominant symptoms often relate to coexisting extra-renal vascular disease (e.g. intermittent claudication).

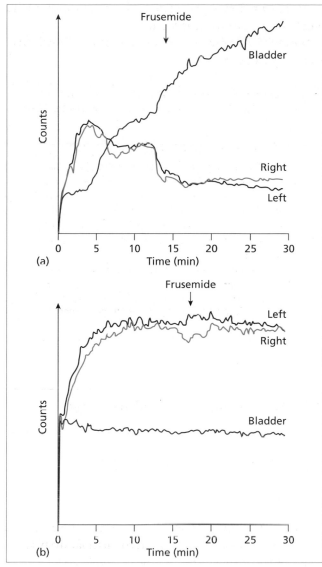

Fig. 80 Captopril renography in the detection of functionally significant bilateral renal artery stenosis. (a) Precaptopril renogram shows normal time-to-peak (<5 min). (b) Postcaptopril renogram shows prolonged time-to-peak and marked cortical retention of isotope in both kidneys.

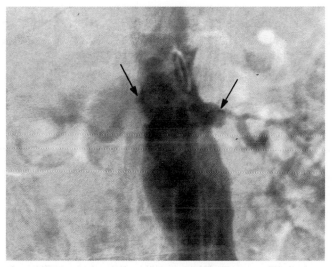

Fig. 81 Aortic aneurysm in association with atheromatous renovascular disease. An infrarenal aneurysm with bilateral renal artery stenoses (arrowed) are shown on this intravenous digital subtraction angiogram (DSA).

- Complicated lesions (e.g. related to aortic aneurysm) may be treated surgically.
- Transplantation is rarely an option because of widespread arterial disease.
- Patients should receive aspirin and cholesterol-lowering therapy for their general atherosclerotic risk, and hypertension should be controlled.

Prognosis

This is poor as a result of co-morbid vascular events; 5-year survival rate on dialysis is less than 20%.

1 Kalra PA. Atherosclerotic renovascular disease. In: *Horizons in Medicine*, No. 11 (Pusey C, ed.). London: Royal College of Physicians of London, 1999: 309–324.
2 Conlon PJ, O'Riordan E, Kalra PA. New insights into the epidemiologic and clinical manifestations of atherosclerotic renovascular disease. *Am J Kidney Dis* 2000; 35: 573–587.

Investigations

- Screening can be with captopril renography (Fig. 80), which has a low sensitivity in patients with CRF, or magnetic resonance imaging
- Doppler ultrasonography is time-consuming and highly observer dependent
- Definitive investigation remains renal angiography (Fig. 81).

Treatment

- Some patients are suitable for renal revascularization with angioplasty with or without stenting, the latter being particularly beneficial for ostial lesions. A successful result is stabilization of CRF [2].

2.5.2 CHOLESTEROL ATHEROEMBOLIZATION

Pathophysiology

Cholesterol crystals embolize to the kidneys and to other distal vessels (e.g. to the feet and skin). They occlude the intrarenal circulation (usually at arteriolar level), resulting in ischaemic renal injury. Occasionally, larger emboli occlude large vessels and lead to infarction [1].

Clinical presentation

Presentation is ARF, particularly complicating intra-arterial angiography and aortic aneurysm surgery. Unlike

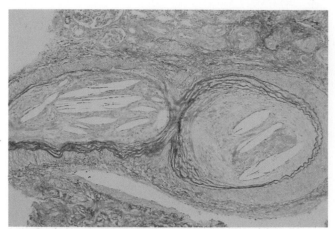

Fig. 82 Intrarenal cholesterol emboli. Large cholesterol crystals are seen within renal arterioles (H&E, ×120).

radiocontrast nephropathy (in which the peak ARF occurs in 1–3 days, with evidence of recovery at 5 days), the ARF persists for many days after the onset, and end-stage renal failure may supervene. Systemic anticoagulation can precipitate emboli. Cholesterol emboli probably contribute to the CRF seen in some patients with ARVD.

Physical signs

There is evidence of generalized atherosclerotic disease in 90%; livedo reticularis (35%) and peripheral cyanosis (Fig. 24, 'trash feet') are commonly seen.

Investigations

Renal biopsy shows typical intra-arteriolar cholesterol crystals (Fig. 82), but changes are patchy and may be missed as a result of sampling error.

Treatment

There are anecdotal reports of clinical improvement accompanying statin therapy. When anticoagulation is implicated, it should be withdrawn if possible. Angiography should be avoided.

Prognosis

Prognosis is poor because of underlying vascular disease. CRF may stabilize if precipitating factors can be removed. Some patients with ARF never recover renal function.

1 Fine MJ, Kapoor W, Falanga V. Cholesterol crystal embolization: a review of 221 cases in the English literature. *Angiology* 1987; 38: 769–784.

2.6 Postrenal problems

2.6.1 OBSTRUCTIVE UROPATHY

Aetiology/pathophysiology/pathology

Obstruction can arise at any point along the urinary tract (Fig. 83). If pressure rises proximal to the obstruction, then the GFR will fall and renal damage may occur.

Obstruction can arise from:
- within the lumen of the urinary tract (e.g. stones)
- within the wall of the system (e.g. urothelial tumours)
- outside the system (e.g. pressure from a pelvic tumour).

Epidemiology

Lower tract obstruction is common in elderly people, mainly in older men with prostatic disease.

Clinical presentation

Acute obstruction, especially with stones, can cause severe pain in the areas to which the urinary tract refers pain—from the loin down to the external genitalia (see Section 1.13, pp. 38–40).

Chronic obstruction is often asymptomatic until there is substantial renal impairment. A poor urinary stream suggests significant obstruction in prostatic disease: hesitancy, terminal dribbling and urinary frequency also occur.

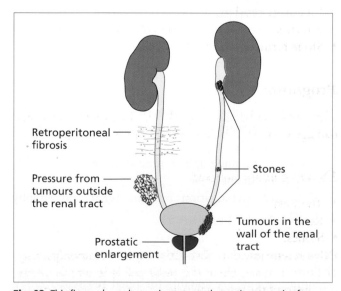

Fig. 83 This figure shows how urinary tract obstruction can arise from outside the wall of the urinary tract, within the wall or within the lumen of the urinary system. The major sites at which obstruction to the urinary tract can occur are shown.

Always consider prostatic obstruction in an older man with renal impairment or urinary tract infection.

 Sacks SH, Aparicio SA, Bevan A, Oliver DO, Will EJ, Davison AM. Late renal failure due to prostatic outflow obstruction: a preventable disease. *BMJ* 1989; 298: 156–159.

Physical signs

- Prostate enlargement
- Large palpable residual bladder volume
- Note that urinary obstruction does not cause the kidneys to become palpable.

Investigation

- Imaging of the renal tract, usually by ultrasonography
- Further imaging to define site and nature of obstruction
- Plasma: evidence of renal impairment
- Specific tests may be relevant, such as prostate-specific antigen.

Differential diagnosis

The differential diagnosis is from other causes of renal impairment.

Treatment

- Surgical or radiological relief of obstruction
- Endocrine treatment of benign prostatic disease with 5α-reductase inhibitors may be of some benefit.

Complications

- End-stage renal disease
- Infection
- Stone formation in static urine.

Prognosis

The renal prognosis depends on the amount of renal damage caused by the obstruction before it is relieved.

Disease associations

- Tumours
- Retroperitoneal fibrosis
- Stones.

Pelviureteric junction obstruction: quite commonly a ring of fibrous tissue where the renal pelvis joins the ureter can obstruct the renal pelvis and calyces. This can correct spontaneously but, if there is pain or evidence of declining renal function, surgery is needed.

2.6.2 STONES

Aetiology/pathophysiology/pathology

Stones form when the concentration of stone-forming substances in the urine exceeds their solubility.

Conditions that raise urinary concentrations of stone-forming substances or lower urinary levels of stone-inhibiting compounds therefore predispose to stones. In particular, if the urine volume is reduced, the concentration of stone-forming substances rises and stone formation increases. Compounds such as citrate reduce stone formation by chelating stone substances.

Hypercalciuria occurs in 65% of patients with stones and is usually idiopathic. It is associated with obesity and hypertension. Major causes of stone formation are shown in Table 23.

Table 23 Major causes of stone formation.

Stone type	Causes
Calcium stones (80%)	• hypercalciuria: causes of hypercalcaemia, especially primary hyperparathyroidism; idiopathic • hyperoxaluria: primary hyperoxaluria; excess intake; ileal disease and ileal bypass • hypocitraturia: distal tubular disease
Uric acid stones (10%)	• acid urine causes uric-acid precipitation • high purine intake • high cell turnover—tumours and tumour lysis
Cystine stones (2%)	• cystinuria—autosomal recessive defect in dibasic amino-acid transporter
Infection stones (5%)	• chronic infection with urea-splitting organisms causes stones made of magnesium ammonium phosphate and calcium phosphate
Other stones (3%)	• include xanthine stones in xanthinuria • rare renal chloride channel mutations can cause stone formation

 Major sites of stone obstruction in the ureters are at:
- The pelviureteric junction
- The point where the ureters cross over the rim of the pelvic bones
- The entry site of the ureters into the bladder.

Epidemiology

Stones are common, with a prevalence of up to 10% in men and 5% in women.

Clinical presentation

The clinical presentation varies:
• Asymptomatic haematuria, uncomplicated passage of small stones or gravel
• Acute renal colic with loin pain, nausea, vomiting and sometimes frank haematuria (see Section 1.13, pp. 38–40).

Physical signs

Obstruction may cause renal tenderness.

Investigations

• Urine: microscopic or macroscopic blood
• Imaging by plain radiography, ultrasonography or contrast studies: calcium and infection stones are radio-opaque, cystine stones are weakly radio-opaque and urate stones are radio-lucent
• Culture urine to exclude infection
• Further investigations may identify a predisposing metabolic disorder: these include biochemical analysis of stones, urine and plasma.

Differential diagnosis

• Clot retention
• Papillary necrosis
• Tumours.

Treatment

Asymptomatic stones not associated with obstruction or infection require conservative treatment only (see Prevention). Symptomatic, obstructing or large stones may be removed by percutaneous or surgical intervention, or by extracorporeal shock wave lithotripsy.

Complications

• Infection
• Urinary obstruction
• Permanent renal damage.

Prognosis

Fifty per cent of those who pass a urinary stone will do so again. Untreated or repeated obstruction can cause chronic renal failure, most commonly with infection stones.

Prevention

Prevention of stone recurrence is by:
• All stones: maintain high fluid intake to keep urinary concentration of stone-forming substances low. Eradicate (if possible) any chronic infection. Potassium citrate is helpful in most stone-forming situations because, as well as alkalinization, the citrate chelates calcium.
• Calcium stones; correct hyperparathyroidism if present. Avoid excesses of animal protein, oxalate-containing foods or calcium intake, but do not advise avoidance of dairy products. Thiazide diuretics can inhibit calcium excretion.
• Urate stones: alkalinization of the urine with potassium citrate or sodium bicarbonate. Reduce purine intake. Allopurinol.
• Cystine stones: alkalinization of the urine. D–penicillamine, which cleaves cystine to soluble cysteine products.

 Borghi L, Meschi T, Schianchi T *et al*. Urine volume: stone risk factor and preventive measure. *Nephron* 1999; 81 (suppl 1): 31–37.

2.6.3 RETROPERITONEAL FIBROSIS OR PERIAORTITIS

Aetiology/pathophysiology/pathology

This is an autoimmune periaortitis, possibly triggered by material leaking out of atheromatous plaques. Histologically there is atheroma, thinning of the media, increased adventitia and inflammatory infiltration of the vessel wall. The lower and mid-thirds of the ureters become embedded in fibrous tissue and can become obstructed.

Epidemiology

• Peak age = 50–70 years
• M : F = 3 : 1.

Clinical presentation

This is with flank or abdominal pain, or as an incidental finding when investigating impaired renal function or vascular disease.

Physical signs

There may be hypertension and signs of vascular disease.

Investigations

• Computed tomography or magnetic resonance imaging (MRI)
• A raised ESR and a normochromic/normocytic anaemia are common
• IVU or retrograde contrast studies may show characteristic medial deviation of the ureters.

Differential diagnosis

- Other causes of urinary tract obstruction
- Malignancy with obstruction.

Treatment

Steroids reduce inflammation and, if still necessary, the ureters can be stented or surgically freed from the fibrotic tissue (ureterolysis).

Prognosis

With treatment the prognosis for renal function is good.

Disease associations

This disease can be triggered by methysergide, and possibly by β-blockers and methyldopa.

Demko TM, Diamond JR, Graff J. Obstructive nephropathy as a result of retroperitoneal fibrosis: a review of its pathogenesis and associations. *J Am Soc Nephrol* 1997; 8: 684–688.

2.6.4 URINARY TRACT INFECTION

Aetiology/pathophysiology/pathology

Infection usually enters the urinary tract through the urethra, but blood-borne infection can deposit in the kidney. The higher incidence in women is attributed to easier access for pathogens through the shorter female urethra.

- The usual organisms are Gram-negative *Escherichia coli*, *Klebsiella* and *Proteus* species
- Lower urinary tract infection is restricted to the bladder and urethra; it usually involves only the superficial mucosa and has no long-term effects
- Upper urinary tract infection, affecting the kidney or ureters, involves the deep renal medullary tissue and can permanently damage the kidney.

During pregnancy, the ureters are relatively dilated and have a lower tone, which increases the risk of infection ascending to the kidneys.

Infection of the urinary tract by *Mycobacterium tuberculosis* is uncommon in the UK but is a cause of sterile pyuria (white cells in the urine, but no organism grown in standard culture conditions). Early morning urine samples should be cultured specifically for mycobacteria when this diagnosis is considered.

Epidemiology

Urinary tract infection is common in all societies.

Clinical presentation

- Variable: asymptomatic bacteriuria, acute uncomplicated lower urinary tract infection, acute pyelonephritis
- Lower tract infection can produce discomfort or burning on micturition, increased urinary frequency and offensive smelling urine
- Upper tract infection can produce loin pain, fever, flank tenderness and rigors.

Physical signs

- Fever
- Tenderness over the kidneys or bladder.

Investigations

- Urinary microscopy and culture: organisms may not be seen, but white cells suggest infection; white cell casts suggest upper tract infection
- If upper tract infection is suspected, take blood cultures.
- In recurrent infection, imaging of the renal tract should be performed to exclude a physical cause, such as stones or partial obstruction.

Differential diagnosis

For acute pyelonephritis, consider renal colic caused by stones and renal infarction.

Treatment

Treatment should involve maintenance of a high fluid intake. Drug therapy should be based on microbiological sensitivities if available:
- For lower tract infection a short course of amoxycillin or trimethoprim is usually curative
- For upper tract infection antibiotics may need to be continued for up to 6 weeks.

Complications

- Septicaemia
- Renal damage
- Stone formation
- Papillary necrosis.

Prognosis

The prognosis is good with treatment.

Prevention

For recurrent urinary tract infection, treat any underlying cause, e.g. remove stones. Women with recurrent infection should be encouraged to void frequently, practise double-micturition (to ensure that the bladder is empty after voiding), and void before and after sexual activity. Long-term prophylactic antimicrobials, e.g. trimethoprim 100 mg at night, may be helpful.

Disease associations

• Pregnancy and anatomical abnormalities, including polycystic kidney disease, stones
• Vesicoureteric reflux: the reflux usually resolves during childhood, but renal damage often happens early in life before this resolution (see Section 2.4.4, pp. 83–86).

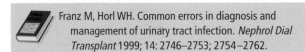

Franz M, Horl WH. Common errors in diagnosis and management of urinary tract infection. *Nephrol Dial Transplant* 1999; 14: 2746–2753; 2754–2762.

2.7 The kidney in systemic disease

2.7.1 MYELOMA

Pathology

The most characterstic finding is intratubular casts (Fig. 84), but glomerular lesions, amyloidosis or chronic interstitial nephritis can also be seen on renal biopsy.

Pathophysiology

In light-chain nephropathy, free κ or λ light chains excreted in the urine damage the tubules by direct nephrotoxicity and cast formation. The intratubular casts composed of hard, needle-shaped crystals excite an interstitial infiltrate, often with multi-nucleate giant cells (Fig. 84). ATN and tubular atrophy occur.

Epidemiology

Acute renal failure occurs in about 5% of those with myeloma; the prevalence of myeloma patients on dialysis programmes is about 2% [1].

Clinical presentation

Acute renal failure is usually associated with light-chain nephropathy; hypercalcaemia, hyperuricaemia, sepsis and

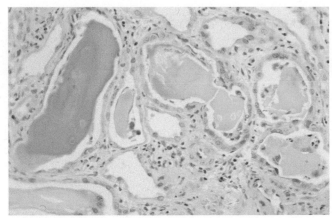

Fig. 84 Myeloma kidney. Dense intratubular casts are shown, with accompanying tubular cell atrophy (H&E, ×200).

radiocontrast agents may also contribute. Myeloma-related amyloid usually presents with CRF and/or the nephrotic syndrome.

Treatment

• ARF may be reversed by vigorous rehydration, treatment of hypercalcaemia and sepsis (see Section 1.14, pp. 40–41), and chemotherapy specific for the myeloma
• Most cases of myeloma presenting with subacute or chronic renal failure progress to end-stage renal failure despite chemotherapy
• Renal transplantation is not appropriate, but dialysis should not be withheld unless the patient is terminally ill.

Prognosis

Prognosis is poor as a result of the underlying myeloma; most patients die from sepsis.

1 Ronco PM, Aucouturier P, Mougenot B. Kidney involvement in plasma cell dyscrasias. In: Davison AM, Cameron JS, Grünfeld J-P, Kerr DNS, Ritz E, Winearls CG (eds) *Oxford Textbook of Clinical Nephrology* (2nd edn). Oxford: Oxford University Press, 1998: 811–835.

2.7.2 AMYLOIDOSIS

Aetiology

There is amorphous deposition of amyloid proteins in the tissues. Amyloidosis is classified according to the amyloid proteins involved (Table 24).

Clinical presentation

Renal amyloid presents with proteinuria, nephrotic syndrome or CRF.

Table 24 Classification of amyloidosis [2].

Type of amyloid	Amyloid protein involved	Underlying cause
Primary amyloid	AL type, which is serum amyloid protein P coupled with immunoglobulin light chains	Plasma cell dyscrasia
Secondary amyloid	This is usually AA type (fibrils composed of acute phase protein)	Secondary to chronic suppurative disorders: • Tuberculosis • Osteomyelitis • Empyema • Bronchiectasis • Syphilis • Leprosy Secondary to chronic inflammatory disorders: • Rheumatoid arthritis • Psoriatic arthritis • Ankylosing spondylitis • Still's disease • Reiter's syndrome • Sjögren's syndrome • Behçet's disease • Whipple's disease • Inflammatory bowel disease • Myeloma (AL type) Other secondary amyloid: • Heroin abuse • Paraplegia • Renal-cell carcinoma
Hereditary amyloid (e.g. Familial Mediterranean Fever)	Fibrils are formed from other proteins (lysozymes, apolipoproteins, fibrinogen)	Abnormal protein
Dialysis-related amyloid	Caused by β2-microglobulin	High circulating levels

Investigation

• Renal ultrasonography demonstrates normal-size or enlarged, echogenic kidneys
• Renal biopsy demonstrates extracellular fibrillar material within the mesangium, interstitium and vessel walls that stains characteristically with Congo red (Fig. 85)
• A serum amyloid P scan may be useful to demonstrate the extent of disease involvement.

Treatment

• AL amyloid may respond to cytotoxic therapy, and there are reports of complete remission with high-dose chemotherapy and stem-cell autotransplantation
• Progression of secondary amyloid can be slowed by control of the underlying inflammatory or infective process [1]
• Liver transplantation can cure familial Mediterranean fever.

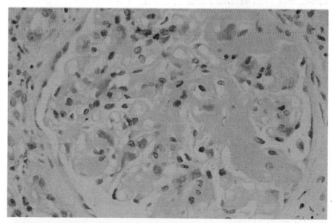

Fig. 85 Renal amyloidosis. Renal biopsy specimen showing diffuse material staining with Congo red within the glomeruli; the patient had had rheumatoid arthritis for 25 years (H&E, ×250).

Prognosis

Patients with end-stage renal failure caused by amyloid have a poor prognosis, the 5-year survival rate being <50% on dialysis; this is usually the result of progressive amyloid in other organs (e.g. cardiomyopathy).

1 Gertz MA, Kyle RA. Secondary systemic amyloidosis: Response and survival in 64 patients. *Medicine* 1991; 70: 246–256.
2 Modified from Kalra PA. Nephrology. In: *Essential Revision Notes for MRCP* (Kalra PA, ed.). Knutsford: Pastest, 1999: 387–438.

2.7.3 HAEMOLYTIC–URAEMIC SYNDROME

Pathology

- Intraglomerular thrombi with ischaemia (Fig. 86)
- Arteriolar lesions.

Epidemiology

Children aged <4 years account for 90% of cases. Two forms of haemolytic–uraemic syndrome (HUS) are recognized:
- The most common form is epidemic, diarrhoea-associated HUS with ARF. A third of UK cases are caused by verotoxin-producing *E. coli* (VTEC); the toxin damages vascular endothelium.
- The sporadic or 'atypical' form tends to affect older children and adults and is not associated with diarrhoea.

A familial form of HUS is described.

Clinical presentation

Presentation is with ARF (it is the most common cause of ARF in children), associated with severe anaemia and systemic bleeding tendency. Neurological disease and severe hypertension are common in 'atypical' HUS.

Investigation

The haematological abnormalities are characteristic—microangiopathic haemolytic anaemia (MAHA), with anaemia, red blood cell (RBC) fragments, schistocytes, etc.

Treatment

Treatment is with fresh frozen plasma and plasma exchange.

Prognosis

The overall mortality rate is 10%; prognosis is worse in adults and particularly in 'atypical' cases, in which CRF may be insidious and progress to end-stage renal failure.

Neild GH, Barratt TM. Acute renal failure associated with microangiopathy. In: Davison AM, Cameron JS, Grünfeld J-P, Kerr DNS, Ritz E, Winearls CG (eds) *Oxford Textbook of Clinical Nephrology* (2nd edn). Oxford: Oxford University Press, 1998: 1649–1666.

2.7.4 SICKLE CELL DISEASE

Pathophysiology

Homozygous sickle cell disease can cause:
- Glomerular disease (thought to result from hyperfiltration injury in childhood)
- Damage to the renal medulla (from ischaemic papillary necrosis as a result of sickle-related occlusion of the vasa rectae).

Clinical presentation

- Enuresis occurs in about 40% (poor concentrating ability)
- Haematuria, resulting from papillary necrosis, occurs in both homozygotes and sickle cell trait
- CRF in adult homozygotes, especially those aged over 40 years [1]
- Less commonly nephrotic syndrome.

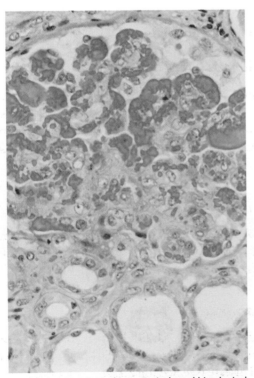

Fig. 86 Haemolytic–uraemic syndrome. Typical renal histological appearance with intraglomerular thrombi (H&E, ×300).

Investigations

IVU may show the 'cup and spill' calyceal deformities of papillary necrosis (Fig. 77). Renal biopsy in CRF demonstrates widespread nephron loss and glomerulosclerosis.

1 Allon M. Renal abnormalities in sickle cell disease. *Arch Intern Med* 1990; 150: 501–504.

2.7.5 AUTOIMMUNE RHEUMATIC DISORDERS

Most autoimmune rheumatic disorders can cause renal disease, but most commonly renal problems are seen in:

- Sjögren's syndrome
- Rheumatoid arthritis
- Systemic sclerosis
- SLE.

Sjögren's syndrome

Pathology

In this there is most frequently an interstitial nephritis.

Clinical presentation

Presentation is with proteinuria, CRF or renal tubular dysfunction, particularly proximal and/or distal RTA.

Treatment

The condition responds to steroids and cyclophosphamide, but these are rarely required for renal manifestations alone.

Rheumatoid arthritis

Pathology

Renal disease may be caused by amyloid, a proliferative glomerulonephritis or the effects of drug therapy [1].

The amyloid is AA. Gold and penicillamine can cause a membranous glomerulonephritis and NSAIDs an interstitial nephritis. A rheumatoid-related mesangioproliferative glomerulonephritis (with IgM deposition) is quite common.

Clinical presentation

Presentation is with proteinuria, nephrotic syndrome (especially amyloid) or renal impairment. Patients with mesangioproliferative glomerulonephritis may have microscopic haematuria.

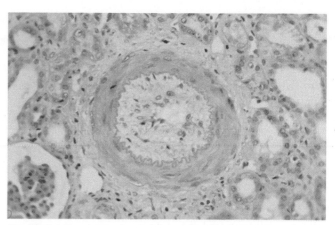

Fig. 87 Vascular changes in scleroderma. Renal biopsy specimen showing obliterative arteriolar lesions with 'onion-skin' appearance and intimal hyperplasia (H&E, ×250).

Treatment

Withdraw offending drugs. Attempt to avoid NSAIDs in all cases of renal impairment (not always possible). As for CRF (Section 2.1.2) and end-stage renal failure (Section 2.1.3).

Prognosis

Patients with amyloidosis usually progress inexorably to end-stage renal failure. Drug-related glomerulonephritis usually resolves within 6 months of withdrawing the agent.

Systemic sclerosis

Pathology

Prominent pathological changes occur in interlobular arteries (severe intimal proliferation with deposition of mucopolysaccharides, forming an 'onion skin'); fibrinoid necrosis of afferent arterioles and secondary glomerular ischaemia are common (Fig. 87).

Clinical presentation

Renal disease is usually accompanied by hypertension. In classic 'scleroderma renal crisis' there is accelerated-phase hypertension, MAHA and ARF [2].

Treatment

Treatment is with ACE inhibitors for control of hypertension. As for CRF (see Section 2.1.2) and end-stage renal disease (see Section 2.1.3).

Prognosis

In many, renal failure is irreversible, but sometimes recovery occurs after months of dialysis. Prognosis is poor because of other organ involvement (especially restrictive cardiomyopathy, pulmonary fibrosis and bowel involvement).

Systemic lupus erythematosus

Pathology

Several patterns of glomerular disease can be seen in SLE (Table 25 and Figs 88 and 89).

Note that in SLE:
• 'Wire-loop' lesions (thickened capillary walls—electron microscopy shows electron-dense deposits) are characteristic (Fig. 89)
• Immunofluorescence is positive for most immunoglobulins (IgG, IgM, IgA) and complement components (C3, C4, C1q).

Epidemiology

Of patients with SLE, 40% have renal involvement at presentation; lupus nephritis is more common in black patients and in women (M : F = 1 : 10).

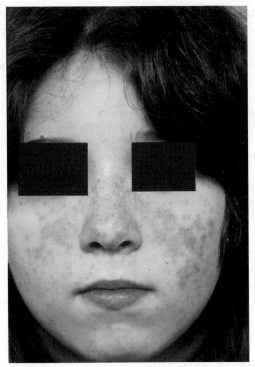

Fig. 88 Typical rash of SLE.

Clinical presentation

Renal disease can be manifest by any syndromal picture, e.g. asymptomatic proteinuria, nephrotic syndrome, ARF.

Treatment

Acute SLE with ARF (usually diffuse or crescentic glomerulonephritis) is treated as for severe renal vasculitis [3].

Table 25 WHO Histological classification of renal involvement in SLE. This classification ignores tubular and interstitial changes which may be better indices of the potential for recovery.

I	minimal change nephropathy	5–10%
II	mesangial glomerulonephritis	10%
III	focal proliferative glomerulonephritis	10%
IV	diffuse proliferative glomerulonephritis (+/− crescents)	50%
V	membranous nephropathy	20%

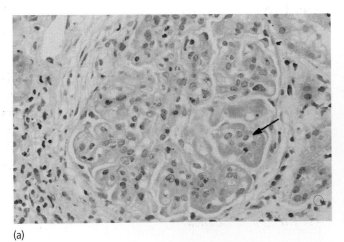

(a)

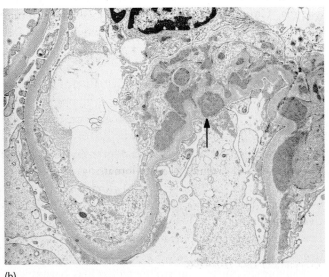

(b)

Fig. 89 Renal histological changes in SLE. (a) Proliferative glomerulonephritis: a typical wire-loop capillary (arrowed) is shown (H&E, ×200). (b) Electron microscopy reveals subendothelial deposits (arrowed) (×20 000).

Other forms of lupus nephritis usually respond to oral steroids with azathioprine, cyclophosphamide, cyclosporin A or mycophenolate mofetil. Randomized trials support the use of oral steroids with intermittent intravenous cyclophosphamide.

As for CRF (see Section 2.1.2) and end-stage renal disease (see Section 2.1.3).

Prognosis

The pattern of renal histological damage is of prognostic value:
• Focal proliferative and membranous lesions have a favourable renal outcome
• Diffuse proliferative or crescentic glomerulonephritis predicts the worst renal prognosis.

See *Rheumatology and clinical immunology*, Section 2.4.2.
1 Emery P, Adu D. Rheumatoid arthritis, mixed connective tissue disease, and polymyositis. In: Davison AM, Cameron JS, Grünfeld J-P, Kerr DNS, Ritz E, Winearls CG (eds) *Oxford Textbook of Clinical Nephrology* (2nd edn). Oxford: Oxford University Press, 1998: 975–985.
2 Shapiro AP, Medsger TA Jr. Renal involvement in systemic sclerosis. In: *Diseases of Kidney*, 4th edn (Schreiner R, Gottschalk C, eds). Boston: Little, Brown, & Co., 1988: 2272–2283.
3 Donadio JV, Glassock RJ. Immunosuppressive drug therapy in lupus nephritis. *Am J Kid Dis* 1993; 21: 239–250.

2.7.6 SYSTEMIC VASCULITIS

In vasculitis, leucocytes damage blood vessels, resulting in tissue ischaemia. The spectrum of disease is wide and depends on the size of the blood vessels affected. The kidney is commonly involved in small vessel vasculitides, often when these are associated with antineutrophil cytoplasmic antibodies (ANCAs), although small vessel vasculitis occurs in other settings, including cryoglobulinaemia, Churg–Strauss syndrome, various autoimmune rheumatic disorders and Henoch–Schönlein purpura (see Section 2.3.1, p. 73).

Pathology

ANCA-associated vasculitis

ANCA-associated vasculitis includes both microscopic polyangiitis and Wegener's granulomatosis.

Renal histology shows necrotizing glomerulitis, typically associated with focal proliferative and/or crescentic glomerulonephritis (Fig. 90). There is little antibody deposition.

Polyarteritis nodosa

This is a medium-sized arterial vasculitis, which classically results in renal infarcts rather than glomerulonephritis.

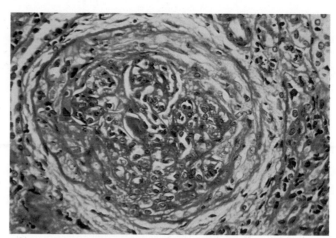

Fig. 90 Crescentic glomerulonephritis. The crescent derives from the epithelial cells of Bowman's capsule (periodic acid–Schiff [PAS], ×300). This appearance is recognized in many forms of aggressive glomerulonephritis, including Goodpasture's disease, ANCA-positive vasculitis and idiopathic rapidly progressive glomerulonephritis.

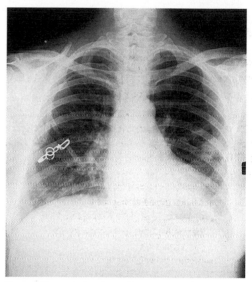

Fig. 91 Chest radiograph showing pulmonary vasculitis in Wegener's granulomatosis. Diffuse infiltrates are seen in the lower zones.

Clinical presentation

ANCA-associated vasculitis

Patients may present with renal failure or systemic manifestations [1]. A purpuric vasculitic skin rash is common. Pulmonary involvement is most frequent in Wegener's granulomatosis, where there may be characteristic necrotizing granulomas in the upper respiratory tract with sinusitis and nasal discharge (Fig. 91). Pulmonary haemorrhage may be life threatening.

Polyarteritis nodosa

Patients can present with ARF, usually associated with severe hypertension. Pulmonary infiltrates and haemorrhage,

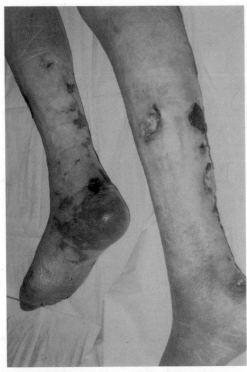

Fig. 92 Vasculitic skin ulcers in polyarteritis nodosa. The ulcers are deep, 'punched-out' and caused by necrosis.

gastrointestinal ischaemia, mononeuritis multiplex, cutaneous vasculitis (Fig. 92) and systemic features (myalgia, pyrexia of unknown origin [PUO]) may occur.

Investigations

ANCA-associated vasculitis

• Microscopic polyangiitis is typically associated with perinuclear ANCA (pANCA) staining directed against myeloperoxidase (MPO). Cytoplasmic ANCA (cANCA) staining can also be seen, directed against proteinase 3 (PR3).
• Wegener's granulomatosis is strongly associated (90% of cases) with cANCA against PR3.

Polyarteritis nodosa

• Patients are usually ANCA negative
• There may be an eosinophilia
• Mesenteric angiography characteristically shows multiple microaneurysms (Fig. 93).
The diagnosis can be difficult to confirm [2].

Treatment

ANCA-associated vasculitis

• Immunosuppressive therapy: generally with corticosteroids and cyclophosphamide initially [3], then maintenance with

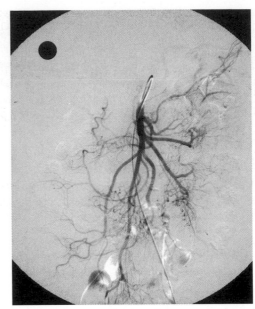

Fig. 93 Mesenteric angiogram showing microaneurysms in polyarteritis nodosa.

tapering steroid doses coupled with azathioprine for at least 2 years
• Role of plasma exchange and pulsed intravenous methylprednisolone not yet defined.

Polyarteritis nodosa

Immunosuppressive regimen similar to that for ANCA-associated vasculitis.

Haworth SJ, Savage COS, Carr D, Hughes JMB, Rees AJ. Pulmonary haemorrhage complicating Wegener's granulomatosis and microscopic polyarteritis. *BMJ* 1985; 290: 355–357.
1 Wilkowski MJ, Velosa JA, Holley KA *et al.* Risk factors in idiopathic renal vasculitis and glomerulonephritis. *Kidney Int* 1989; 36: 133–141.
2 Guillevin L, Le The Huong Du, Godeau P, Jais P, Wechsler B. Clinical findings and prognosis of polyarteritis nodosa and Churg–Strauss angiitis: a study in 165 patients. *Br J Rheum* 1988; 27: 258–264.
3 Pusey CD, Rees AJ. Acute renal failure due to vasculitis and glomerulonephritis. In: Davison AM, Cameron JS, Grünfeld J-P, Kerr DNS, Ritz E, Winearls CG (eds) *Oxford Textbook of Clinical Nephrology* (2nd edn). Oxford: Oxford University Press, 1998: 1060–1076.

2.7.7 DIABETIC NEPHROPATHY

Pathology

Kimmelstiel–Wilson nodules (focal glomerular sclerosis) are characteristic, but mesangial matrix expansion and diffuse glomerular sclerosis with vascular changes are more common (Fig. 94).

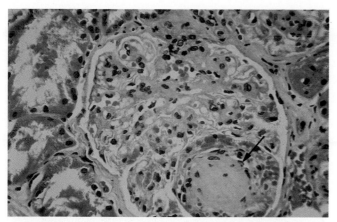

Fig. 94 Diabetic nephropathy. A classic Kimmelstiel–Wilson nodule (arrowed) is present with a background of diffuse mesangial sclerosis (H&E, ×250).

Epidemiology

Diabetic nephropathy is one of the most common causes of end-stage renal failure. About 40% of patients with type 1 diabetes mellitus have nephropathy 20–40 years after diagnosis and about 25% of patients with type 2 diabetes mellitus develop nephropathy [1].

Clinical presentation

- The earliest sign is microalbuminuria (albumin excretion of 20–200 μg/min or 30–300 mg/day), not reliably detected by standard dipstick
- A majority of patients with microalbuminuria will then develop overt diabetic nephropathy with proteinuria >0.5 g/day (Fig. 95), going on to develop hypertension and chronic renal failure, with about 30% becoming nephrotic

- Nephropathy is usually associated with retinopathy (common basement membrane pathology)
- Macrovascular disease is common.

Treatment

- ACE inhibitors can prevent progression from micro-albuminuria to overt nephropathy
- In established nephropathy, excellent blood pressure and glycaemic control may slow progression
- Combined renal and pancreatic transplantation is now feasible in selected patients.

Prognosis

Once there is renal impairment in diabetic nephropathy, decline to end-stage renal failure is usually inexorable. Mortality is high—patients with type 1 diabetes have a 20-fold greater mortality than the general population, and relative risk is increased further in those with proteinuria (e.g. 2-year mortality rate of 30% in patients with end-stage renal failure), largely as a result of cardiovascular disease.

 1 Watts GF, Shaw KM. Diabetic nephropathy. In: *Renal Disease: Prevention and treatment* (Raman GV, Golper TA, eds). London: Chapman & Hall, 1998: 137–171.

2.7.8 HYPERTENSION

The kidney may be damaged by essential hypertension, and is often the cause of secondary hypertension [1]. Important factors include the following:

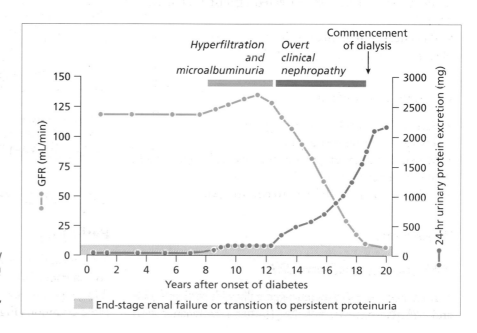

Fig. 95 Clinical course of diabetic nephropathy (in a patient with type 1 diabetes). This schema demonstrates the typical temporal relationship between the development of microalbuminuria, proteinuria and progressive decline in GFR.

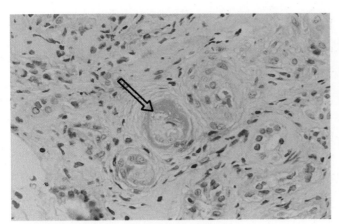

Fig. 96 Accelerated-phase hypertension. Renal histological appearance of 'malignant' hypertension—severe arteriolar lesions include intimal hyperplasia and fibrinoid necrosis (arrowed) of the media (H&E, ×200).

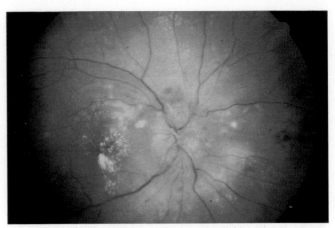

Fig. 97 The retina in accelerated-phase hypertension. There is papilloedema, cotton wool spots and hard retinal exudates, as well as haemorrhage (grade IV hypertensive retinopathy).

• Renin release and activation of the renin–angiotensin–aldosterone axis
• Reduced natriuretic capacity in renal disease
• Disorganization of intrarenal vascular structures.

Pathology

• In essential hypertension, renal damage is manifest by vascular wall thickening and luminal obliteration, with interstitial fibrosis and glomerulosclerosis (hypertensive nephrosclerosis)
• In accelerated-phase hypertension [2], there is arterial fibrinoid necrosis with tubular and glomerular ischaemia (Fig. 96).
• A range of renal pathological conditions can be complicated by hypertension.

Epidemiology

Hypertension affects up to 15% of the population, most of this being 'essential'. Renal disease is the most common cause of secondary hypertension. Of patients approaching end-stage renal failure, 80% are hypertensive.

Clinical presentation

• Patients with essential hypertension may develop proteinuria or CRF (hypertensive nephrosclerosis)
• Accelerated-phase hypertension is a cause of ARF.

Physical signs

• Essential hypertension can cause end-organ damage: heart (left ventricular hypertrophy, cardiac failure); kidneys (proteinuria, increased creatinine); eyes (Grade I and II retinopathy); brain (stroke).
• Accelerated-phase hypertension; characteristic finding is Grade III (haemorrhages and exudates) or IV (with

papilloedema) retinopathy (Fig. 97); also as for essential hypertension.

Investigations

To determine evidence of end-organ damage and look for evidence of a secondary cause, all hypertensive patients should have their serum creatinine and urinalysis checked.

Kincaid-Smith P. Malignant hypertension. *J Hypertension* 1991; 9: 893–899.
1 De Wardener HE. The primary role of the kidney and salt intake in the aetiology of essential hypertension. *Clin Sci* 1990; 79: 193–200.
2 Klahr S. The kidney in hypertension—villain or victim? *N Engl J Med* 1989; 320: 731–733.

2.7.9 SARCOIDOSIS

Epidemiology

Hypercalciuria occurs in 65% of patients and hypercalcaemia in about 20%. Clinically important renal disease is relatively uncommon, although renal impairment has been reported in 15–40%.

Clinical presentation

This is usually with renal impairment in the context of other features of sarcoidosis [1]. Tubular proteinuria, Fanconi's syndrome and distal or proximal RTA are all recognized. Nephrocalcinosis sometimes occurs, but renal calculi are not common.

Investigation

In patients with CRF, renal biopsy usually shows a granulomatous interstitial nephritis (Fig. 98). Sarcoid-related

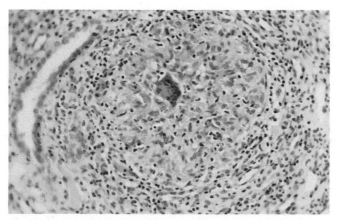

Fig. 98 Sarcoidosis. Typical renal histological appearance with chronic interstitial nephritis and giant-cell granulomatous change (central field) (H&E, ×160).

glomerulopathy (usually membranous glomerulonephritis) is rare.

Treatment

Both hypercalcaemia and interstitial nephritis respond to corticosteroids in moderate dosage.

1 Kenouch S, Mery JP. Sarcoidosis. In: Davison AM, Cameron JS, Grünfeld J-P, Kerr DNS, Ritz E, Winearls CG (eds) *Oxford Textbook of Clinical Nephrology* (2nd edn). Oxford: Oxford University Press, 1998: 837–843.

2.7.10 HEPATORENAL SYNDROME

Pathophysiology

Severe liver disease is associated with marked intrarenal hypoperfusion, probably related to excess of vasoconstrictor mediators. Renal parenchymal damage does not occur and, if transplanted, the kidney will function normally in a recipient with normal liver function.

Epidemiology

Hepatorenal syndrome occurs in about 20% of people with cirrhosis admitted to hospital. It is also common in jaundiced patients requiring major surgery for biliary or pancreatic disease [1].

Clinical presentation

This is of acute renal failure in the context of severe liver disease.

Investigations

Urinary biochemistry shows a very low sodium concentration (<10 mmol/L).

Treatment

Dialysis and other intensive support are appropriate only in patients with potentially remediable liver disease, or candidates for liver transplantation.

Prevention

The mortality of hepatorenal syndrome is high. Prevention in vulnerable patients is important:
- Avoid precipitants, e.g. hypovolaemia
- Identify and treat sepsis
- Ensure intraoperative diuresis (e.g. with mannitol) in patients undergoing surgery.

1 Sweny P. The hepatorenal syndrome. In: *Acute Renal Failure* (Rainford D, Sweny P, eds). London: Farrand Press, 1990: 83–112.

2.7.11 PREGNANCY AND THE KIDNEY

The circulatory and physiological changes of pregnancy affect the kidney:
- GFR increases by up to 50% in the first trimester of normal pregnancy
- The ureters and renal pelvis become more dilated (Fig. 99), the risk of lower urinary tract infection is increased
- Pre-eclampsia is common and involves the kidney, with proteinuria being a feature

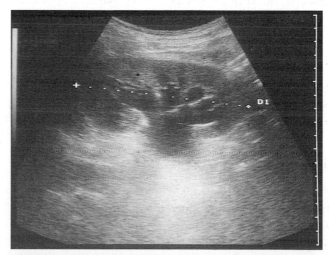

Fig. 99 Hydronephrosis of pregnancy. Typical ultrasonographic appearance.

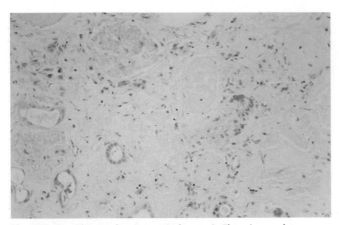

Fig. 100 Renal biopsy showing cortical necrosis. There is complete necrosis of the majority of visible structures (including glomeruli) (H&E, ×160).

• At the time of delivery, placental abruption and severe pre-eclampsia are causes of ARF: irreversible cortical necrosis rather than reversible ATN can occur (Fig. 100).

Chronic renal failure before pregnancy has implications for both fetus and mother (see Section 1.2, pp. 5–7).

Epidemiology

• Asymptomatic bacteriuria in about 5%. If untreated, symptomatic infection develops in about 25% of these
• Pre-eclampsia occurs in 1–2%
• ARF complicates 1 in 6000 pregnancies.

Clinical presentation

This is with urinary infection, pre-eclampsia or ARF. Idiopathic postpartum ARF is associated with severe hypertension and disseminated intravascular coagulation (DIC) [1].

Investigations

Proteinuria most commonly occurs in the context of pre-eclampsia. This typically resolves within 3 months of delivery and requires investigation if it does not.

Peripartum ARF is usually haemodynamically mediated and recovery is anticipated. If this is not forthcoming, renal perfusion can be assessed by radionuclide scan and a biopsy may be appropriate.

Treatment

• Patients with significant bacteriuria should receive antibiotics
• Hypertension should be tightly controlled in pre-eclampsia. Suitable agents include methyldopa, hydralazine, nifedipine and labetalol.

Prognosis

In patients with ARF, the maternal mortality rate is 10–15%. Renal recovery is anticipated in those with ATN, but not in those with cortical necrosis. The perinatal mortality is also very high. In patients with CRF, the chance of a successful pregnancy declines as the GFR falls and is unusual with GFR <20 mL/min [2].

1 Davison JM. Renal complications which can occur in pregnancy. In: Davison AM, Cameron JS, Grünfeld J-P, Kerr DNS, Ritz E, Winearls CG (eds) *Oxford Textbook of Clinical Nephrology* (2nd edn). Oxford: Oxford University Press, 1998: 2317–2325.
2 Davison JM, Baylis C. Pregnancy in patients with underlying renal disease. In: Davison AM, Cameron JS, Grünfeld J-P, Kerr DNS, Ritz E, Winearls, CG (eds) *Oxford Textbook of Clinical Nephrology* (2nd edn). Oxford: Oxford University Press, 1998: 2327–2348.

2.8 Genetic renal conditions

2.8.1 AUTOSOMAL DOMINANT POLYCYSTIC KIDNEY DISEASE

Aetiology/pathophysiology/pathology

There is progressive development of renal cysts (Fig. 101). Two genetic loci have been described:
• *PKD1* on chromosome 16: 85% of cases; encodes polycystin 1, a large transmembrane molecule possibly involved in cell/matrix interactions
• *PKD2* on chromosome 4: 10% of cases; encodes polycystin 2 which may associate with polycystin 1.

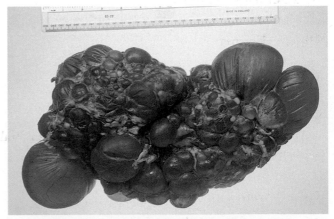

Fig. 101 Macroscopic appearance of a polycystic kidney. (Courtesy of Dr D Peat.)

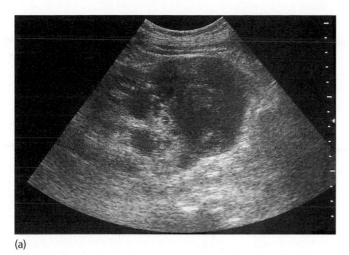

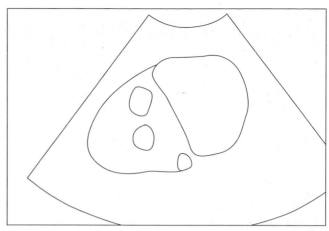

(a)

Fig. 102 Ultrasonogram showing enlarged kidney with multiple cysts.

Epidemiology

- The most common inherited renal disease
- 5–10% of patients with end-stage renal failure
- Prevalence 1 : 400 to 1 : 1000.

Clinical presentation

Common

- 30% acute or chronic abdominal pain
- 20% hypertension
- 20% gross haematuria
- 5–40% urinary tract infection; more common in women
- Incidental discovery of abdominal mass
- Family screening.

Uncommon

End-stage renal failure.

Rare

Intracranial haemorrhage.

Physical signs

Common

- Palpable kidneys and/or liver
- Hypertension
- Murmurs associated with mitral regurgitation or mitral valve prolapse.

Uncommon

Murmurs associated with tricuspid regurgitation or aortic incompetence.

Investigations

Diagnosis by multiple bilateral renal cysts and a positive family history:

- Ultrasonography (Fig. 102): in *PKD1* families, diagnostic criteria are age related (two cysts in <30 years age group, at least two cysts in each kidney in 30–59 years age group and four cysts in each kidney for >60 year olds). Normal ultrasonography after age 30 years (but not before) excludes the diagnosis.
- Computed tomography: more sensitive than ultrasonography and may aid diagnosis in younger patients.
- Genetic linkage studies: can exclude or make the diagnosis in younger patients. Requires blood from at least two affected family members.
- Magnetic resonance angiography (MRA): in patients with a family history of intracranial aneurysm. In other PKD families screening for cerebral aneurysms is controversial.

Other investigations are as for chronic renal disease (see Section 2.1.2, pp. 50–52).

Differential diagnosis

Simple renal cysts.

Treatment

- Antihypertensives reduce cardiovascular complications, but probably do not slow progression of renal disease
- Treat urinary infections; often problematic; cyst drainage can sometimes be required
- Analgesia: occasionally drainage or deroofing of large cysts may give long-term relief in those whose kidneys are painful.

Complications

Common

- End-stage renal failure in about 75% *PKD1*: at about 50–60 years of age, and *PKD2*: at about 65–75 years of age
- Cardiovascular disease associated with hypertension and CRF
- Urinary tract infection
- Bleed into a cyst.

Rare

Ruptured intracranial aneurysm.

Prognosis

This is as for chronic renal failure.

Disease associations

- 20% valvular heart lesions: mitral regurgitation, mitral valve prolapse, tricuspid regurgitation and aortic regurgitation in decreasing order of frequency.
- 8% have intracranial aneurysms.

Important information for patients

Support groups and Internet information are sometimes helpful. Genetic counselling for family members should be discussed.

Demetriou K Tziakouri C, Anninou K *et al.* Autosomal dominant kidney disease—type 2. Ultrasound, genetic and clinical correlations. *Nephrol Dial Transplant* 2000; 15: 205–211.
Ravine D, Gibson RN, Walker RG, Sheffield LJ, Kincaid-Smith P, Danks DM. Evaluation of ultrasonic diagnostic criteria for autosomal dominant polycystic kidney disease 1. *Lancet* 1994; 343: 824–827.

2.8.2 ALPORT'S SYNDROME

Aetiology/pathophysiology/pathology

There is abnormal glomerular basement membrane (GBM) ultrastructure and sensorineural deafness. The defect is in type IV collagen, a key component of the GBM.
- X-linked dominant: 85–90% of cases. Mutations in the *COL4A5* gene coding for the α_5 chain of type IV collagen. Causes exclusion of the α_3 chain which contains the Goodpasture's disease antigen.
- Autosomal recessive: 10% of cases. Similar to X-linked disease but equally severe in females.

- Autosomal dominant: uncommon. Various mutation sites identified.

Epidemiology

- Gene frequency 1 : 5000 to 1 : 10000
- 0.6% of patients on dialysis in Europe have Alport's syndrome.

Clinical presentation

Common

- Microscopic or macroscopic haematuria
- Hearing loss
- Renal impairment.

Physical signs

Common

- High-tone sensorineural hearing loss
- Bilateral anterior lenticonus.

Investigations

- Audiometry
- Slit-lamp examination of eye
- Renal biopsy—electron microscopy: shows GBM structural abnormalities.

Differential diagnosis

- Other causes of haematuria, e.g. IgA nephropathy
- Non-progressive hereditary nephritis
- Other (rare) syndromes with deafness and renal impairment.

Treatment

There is no specific treatment.

Complications

Common

- End-stage renal failure (see Section 2.1.3, p. 56): all boys with the X-linked form progress to end-stage renal failure, usually by 15–30 years. Most females never reach end-stage renal failure but have persistent haematuria and/or proteinuria. Some develop end-stage renal failure at 30–60 years of age.
- Hearing loss is progressive; a hearing aid may be required.

Rare

Spontaneous lens rupture.

Prognosis

This is as for chronic renal disease (see Section 2.1.2, p. 55).

Kashtan CE. Alport syndrome. An inherited disorder of renal, ocular, and cochlear basement membranes. *Medicine (Baltimore)* 1999; 78: 338–360.

2.8.3 X-LINKED HYPOPHOSPHATAEMIC VITAMIN D-RESISTANT RICKETS

Aetiology/pathophysiology/pathology

This is the most common hereditary form of isolated renal phosphate wasting. Hypophosphataemia, together with a functional defect in osteoblasts, leads to abnormal mineralization of growing bone. The defect is in the *PHEX* gene which codes for a Zn metallopeptidase. The pathogenesis is unclear.

Epidemiology

The incidence is 1 : 20000.

Clinical presentation

Common

- Growth delay usually noted by 6 months
- Hypertension
- Rickets which develops after the child starts walking
- Bone pain.

Physical signs

Common

- Small stature
- Rickets mainly affecting the legs.

Investigations

- 24-h urinary phosphate and calcium excretion
- Calcium, phosphate, PTH, 1,25-dihydroxycholecalciferol (1,25-DHCC)
- Urea, creatinine and electrolyte, glucose, bicarbonate.

Expect to see a low serum phosphate with inappropriate phosphaturia. A normal serum calcium, potassium, glucose, bicarbonate and PTH all rule out syndromes with other renal tubular defects or nutritional rickets. 1,25-Dihydroxycholecalciferol is often slightly low.

Treatment

- High-dose 1,25-DHCC
- Oral phosphate supplements: these are often poorly tolerated as a result of associated diarrhoea
- Recombinant growth hormone may reduce growth delay.

Complications

Uncommon

Treatment-associated hypercalcaemia can cause nephrocalcinosis and renal damage.

Prognosis

- Growth rate can be improved, although final stature is usually abnormal
- Females are less severely affected.

Rowe PS. The role of the PHEX gene (PEX) in families with X-linked hypophosphataemic rickets. *Curr Opin Nephrol Hypertens* 1998; 7: 367–376.

3 Investigations and practical procedures

3.1 Examination of the urine

3.1.1 URINALYSIS

Indications

Urinalysis must be performed in all patients with renal disease/dysfunction. In addition, it is appropriate as a screening test in almost any clinical setting because:
- The consequences of renal failure are serious
- Substantial loss of renal function occurs in a wide range of clinical settings with no specific clinical symptoms
- Serious renal disease is virtually excluded if urinalysis is negative and the GFR is normal.

Practical details

Urinalysis for blood and protein provides a sensitive, cheap, non-invasive screening test.

Estimation of protein content

This can be done by a dipstick at the bedside or in the laboratory.

Dipstick for albumin

This is more sensitive to albumin than to other proteins. Threshold for albumin is 150–300 mg/L.

INDICATIONS AND INTERPRETATION

- Screening test for significant albuminuria
- Negative does not exclude immunoglobulin light chain excretion
- Measures concentration, not rate of protein loss; for the same rate of protein loss, concentrations will be lower when urine is dilute (e.g. after loop diuretic)
- Contamination with skin cleanser/antiseptics (e.g. chlorhexidine) can give false-positive results
- Trace results, especially in concentrated urine, are usually not clinically significant
- Positive results should usually be followed by quantitative urine protein determination.

Dipstick for microalbuminuria

In people with diabetes, development of microalbuminuria (20–200 mg/L) identifies a group at high risk of progressive renal failure. This degree of albuminuria is not reliably detected by standard urine dipsticks, but is with antibody (rather than chemical) detection (e.g. Micral-Test II, Roche).

Laboratory determination of protein content

- Used to quantify protein excretion, e.g. after positive dipstick urinalysis
- Methods used are equally sensitive to different proteins—measures total protein concentration (immunoglobulins, light chains, etc. in addition to albumin)
- Can give protein excretion rate from a sample of known volume, produced over a known time
- Alternatively, protein excretion rate can be predicted from protein/creatinine ratio (avoiding need for timed collections) because creatinine excretion is about 8.8 mmol/day per 1.73 m^2.

Testing for haem

Urine dipstick threshold is 150 μg haemoglobin per litre—equivalent to 5000 red cells/mL.
- Will give positive test with red cells, haemoglobin or myoglobin
- A negative test effectively excludes the presence of abnormal numbers of red cells in the urine.

All people excrete some red cells in their urine, hence positive tests are common—2.5–4% of healthy adult men in population-based studies. The possibility that these results could be caused by serious renal or urological disease (e.g. transitional cell carcinoma) should always be considered (see Section 1.1).

 Intact red cells will sediment on centrifugation, whereas haemoglobin or myoglobin will not. In haemoglobinuria or myoglobinuria, the supernatant will remain pink/red and positive on dipstick testing, whereas in haematuria it will not (Fig. 103).

Other selected urine tests

- Urinalysis for nitrites: screening test for urine infection

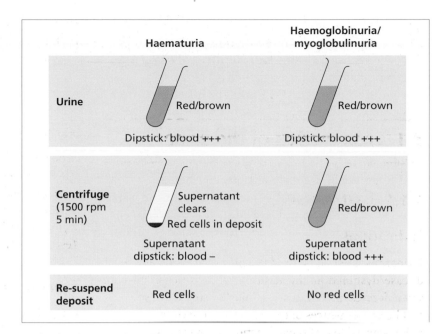

Fig. 103 Distinguishing haematuria (red cells in urine) from haemoglobinuria/myoglobinuria.

• Urinalysis for leucocytes: screening for infection; also positive when white cells present in sterile urine (e.g. interstitial nephritis)
• Urinalysis for glucose: glucose present if lowered renal threshold for glucose or elevated blood glucose concentration
• Urine sodium content: 24-h excretion useful in assessing sodium intake; can be useful in establishing that renal failure is prerenal
• Urine osmolality: used in diagnosis of diabetes insipidus, syndrome of inappropriate secretion of antidiuretic hormone (SIADH)
• Urine pH: diagnosis of RTA; monitor in situations where particular urine pH desirable (e.g. preventing urate deposition in tumour lysis)
• Urine electrophoresis: for light chains (Bence Jones protein)
• Urine calcium, oxalate and citrate determination in those with stones.

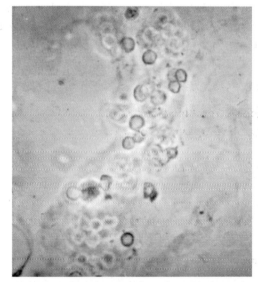

Fig. 104 Red cell cast from the urine of a patient with glomerulonephritis, viewed with phase contrast.

3.1.2 URINE MICROSCOPY

Principle

• Centrifuge 10 mL urine at 1500 rev/min for 5 min, sedimenting cellular elements, casts, crystals
• Re-suspend sediment in 1 mL (may also stain)
• View under microscope.
Red cell casts are particularly important in establishing that there is glomerular inflammation (Fig. 104).

Indications

• Reduced GFR
• Abnormality on dipstick urinalysis.

3.2 Estimation of glomerular filtration rate

Principle

An ideal marker for GFR would have the following characteristics:
• Steady-state level in plasma
• Glomerulus represents no barrier to filtration
• No tubular absorption or secretion
• No extrarenal clearance.

GFR = ([Concentration in urine] × [Urine production rate]) / [Concentration in plasma]

Accurate determinations for research and certain clinical purposes are based on administration of inulin, or labelled ethylenediaminetetra-acetic acid (EDTA) or diethylenetriaminepenta-acetic acid (DTPA).

In routine practice, GFR can be predicted from measurements of creatinine. There is some tubular secretion in addition to glomerular filtration, and also extrarenal clearance of about 2 mL/min. Creatinine clearance (determined accurately) therefore tends to be an overestimate of GFR, especially as renal function deteriorates.

Production is influenced by diet and lean muscle mass. Those who are smaller, older and on a low-protein diet will have lower plasma creatinine for the same creatinine clearance.

Practical details

Timed urine collection

The problem is timing and completeness of urine collection. The total amount of creatinine in the urine collection gives a guide to this. In adults aged <50 years, creatinine production should be 175–220 μmol/kg lean body weight (men) and 135–175 μmol/kg (women). From age 50 to 90 years, this falls by 50%. In a particular patient, if diet and muscle mass remain stable, creatinine excretion from one collection to another will be unchanged.

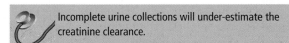 Incomplete urine collections will under-estimate the creatinine clearance.

Estimations based on age, sex and weight

If plasma creatinine is stable, the creatinine clearance can be estimated using empirically derived formulae (see below), whose main advantage is that they avoid the problem of timed urine collections, and are based on a readily available blood test.

 Prediction of creatinine clearance from plasma creatinine
These equations [1] can be misleading in very obese patients, or if there is extensive oedema or ascites.
- For males:
CrCl (mL/min) = [(140 − Age in years) × Weight (kg)] × 1.23 / [Plasma creatinine (μmol/L)]
- For females:
CrCl (mL/min) = [(140 − Age in years) × Weight (kg)] × 1.04 / [Plasma creatinine (μmol/L)]

 Plasma creatinine will be normal (for a short time) even if there is no glomerular filtration! In acute renal failure creatinine will be accumulating rapidly in the plasma, but this cannot be discerned from a single value. GFR can be predicted only if the plasma creatinine is stable.

 1 Cockcroft DW, Gault MH. Prediction of creatinine clearance from serum creatinine. *Nephron* 1976; 16: 31–41.

3.3 Imaging the renal tract

By far the most commonly used method is ultrasonography, which is cheap, reliable and non-invasive. Other tests are used in specific clinical settings.

Ultrasonography

This should be performed in all those with reduced GFR or abnormal urinary findings.

Important findings on ultrasonography include the following:
- Renal size (Fig. 105)
- Obstruction (Fig. 106)

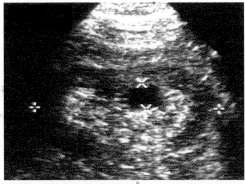

Fig. 105 Ultrasonogram of the kidney in chronic renal failure. The length is reduced (8.15 cm), the cortex thinned and there is a simple cyst (1.1 cm).

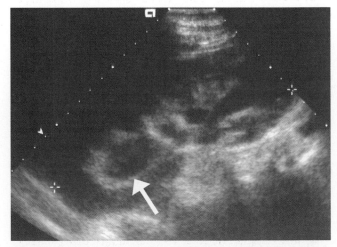

Fig. 106 Ultrasonogram of an obstructed kidney. Length is enlarged at 14 cm. Calyces are dilated (arrow). Cortical thickness is preserved.

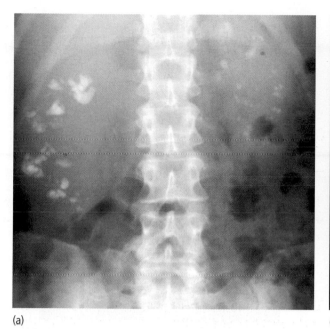
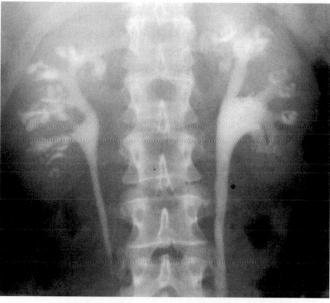

(a)   (h)

Fig. 107 (a) Plain abdominal radiograph and (b) IVU of a patient with medullary sponge kidney with marked nephrocalcinosis.

- Scars (reflux pyelonephritis)
- Cysts (autosomal dominant polycystic kidney disease [ADPKD])
- Renal tumours
- Renal stones
- Thickness of renal cortex.

 Occasionally obstruction is not evident on ultrasonography—usually when it has occurred rapidly, recently and the patient is volume depleted. If there is a high index of suspicion, repeat the ultrasonography after correcting the volume depletion. Negative ultrasound findings can also occur when obstruction is caused by malignant encasement of the kidneys.

Plain abdominal radiograph

This is useful in detecting calculi and nephrocalcinosis (Fig. 107a). Distinction of ureteric stones from phleboliths may require IVU.

Intravenous urography

Radiographic contrast medium is injected, which is filtered by the glomerulus and concentrated in the tubule. The contrast medium is radio-opaque and is visible on radiographs as it passes through the kidney, ureter and bladder (Fig. 107b).

Indications

- In many circumstances, IVU is superseded by ultrasonography and/or cross-sectional imaging

- Useful mainly for imaging the ureters (e.g. for stones or transitional cell carcinoma) which are not reliably visualized on ultrasonography
- Also useful in demonstrating renal scars.

Contraindications

- Sensitivity to contrast agents
- Less informative as GFR falls because clearance and concentration of the contrast medium are reduced.

Retrograde ureterography

Radiographic contrast medium is injected into the ureter from below, using a cystoscope (Fig. 108). This technique is indicated for imaging the ureter when GFR is too low for IVU to be useful.

Isotopic imaging

The following compounds are often used:
- ^{99m}Tc-dimercaptosuccinic acid (DMSA): filtered by the glomerulus and then taken up by the tubules. Useful in detecting renal scars (particularly in children).
- ^{99m}Tc-mercaptoacetyltriglycine (MAG$_3$): secreted by the tubules.
- ^{99m}Tc-DTPA: filtered by the glomerulus.

Indications

- Detection of renal scars: DMSA—screening children with suspected reflux nephropathy or UTI for scars. More sensitive than IVU.

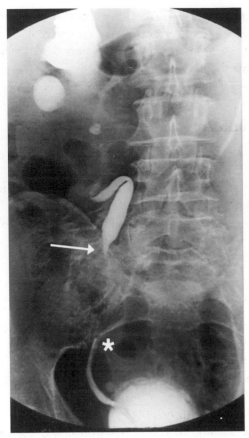

Fig. 108 Retrograde ureterogram. A catheter is inserted in the lower ureter from the bladder (*). Contrast outlines a tapered stricture (arrow) and the obstructed calyceal system.

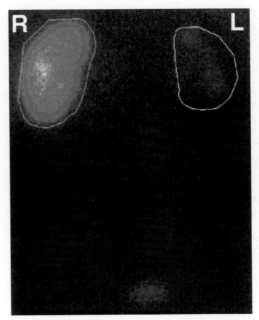

Fig. 109 DMSA scintigraphy of the kidneys. The left kidney is not seen because it is non-functioning: it was subsequently removed.

- Assessment of contribution to GFR of each kidney: DMSA or DTPA scan, e.g. before nephrectomy (Fig. 109).
- Screening for renal artery stenosis: DTPA or MAG$_3$. Sensitivity enhanced by administration of captopril 1 hour previously. Renal artery stenosis indicated by decreased, delayed uptake by one kidney. Not useful if GFR substantially reduced.

Computed tomography

- Evaluation of space-occupying lesions in the kidney or requirement for detailed anatomical knowledge (Fig. 110)
- Investigation of extrinsic problems impinging on the renal tract (e.g. ureteric compression in retroperitoneal fibrosis)
- Spiral computed tomography can be used to examine the renal arteries.

Renal angiography

- Establish anatomy of renal vessels in living kidney donors
- Diagnosis of renal artery stenosis and fibromuscular hyperplasia (Fig. 111a)

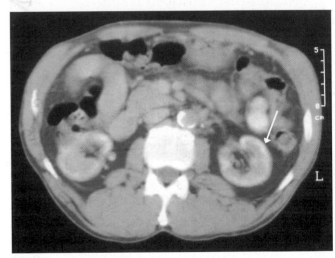

Fig. 110 A CT scan of the abdomen without contrast showing calcification of the renal cortex. This patient had acute cortical necrosis during an episode of acute pancreatitis.

- Establish (and potentially embolize) site of bleeding in the kidney, e.g. after renal biopsy or percutaneous nephrostomy (Fig. 111b)
- Renal venography (or venous phase of intra-arterial digital subtraction angiography [DSA]): to diagnose renal vein thrombosis.

Magnetic resonance imaging

This is a likely method of choice for evaluation of many space-occupying lesions and for imaging the renal artery and vein.

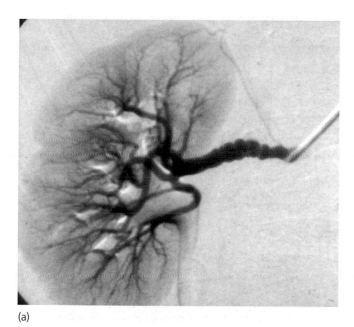

(a)

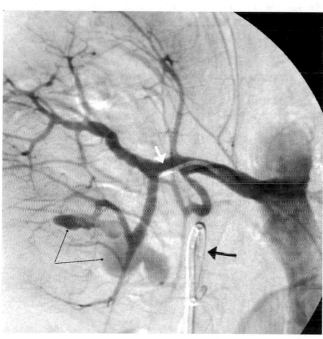

(b)

Fig. 111 (a) Renal angiogram showing fibromuscular hyperplasia. (b) Renal angiogram showing a fistula from the renal circulation into the pelvicalyceal system after percutaneous nephrostomy. A catheter is seen in the renal artery (white arrow). Also seen is the upper end of a ureteric stent (heavy black arrow). Contrast is seen to enter the dilated pelvicalyceal system (fine black arrows). The fistula was successfully embolized with resolution of haematuria.

3.4 Renal biopsy

Principle

Needle biopsies of the kidney are taken and processed as follows (Fig. 112):

- Paraffin: for H&E (haematoxylin and eosin) staining and special stains (e.g. silver stain, Congo red)
- Frozen sections: immunofluorescence for immunoglobulins, complement components
- Resin embedding: for electron microscopy.

Indications

- Investigation of unexplained acute and chronic renal disease
- Most frequently useful in the diagnosis of glomerular disease
- Should be performed only if the result could alter management
- Expert renal histology must be available.

Contraindications

These are relative, rather than absolute. The decision will depend on the clinical setting.
- Single kidney: possibility of losing the kidney
- Reduced renal size: less likely to be diagnostic, more likely to bleed
- Difficulty breath-holding
- Hypertension: increased risk of haemorrhage; should be corrected before biopsy
- Reduced platelet count, reduced haematocrit, abnormal coagulation tests: increase risk of haemorrhage. Should be corrected before biopsy.

Practical details

Before the investigation

- Ultrasonography or other formal imaging defining number, size, localization of kidneys
- FBC, coagulation screen, group and save
- Appropriate premedication
- In severe renal impairment, consider DDAVP infusion (raises levels of von Willebrand factor and factor VIII, ameliorates bleeding tendency related to uraemia).

The investigation

1 The patient lies prone.
2 The lower pole of the kidney is localized using ultrasonography.
3 The kidney moves down with inspiration, and the operator directs the patient's respiration.
4 A spinal needle is used to anaesthetize the track, and to localize the kidney. It is advanced forward only when the patient holds their breath so that the kidney is stationary.

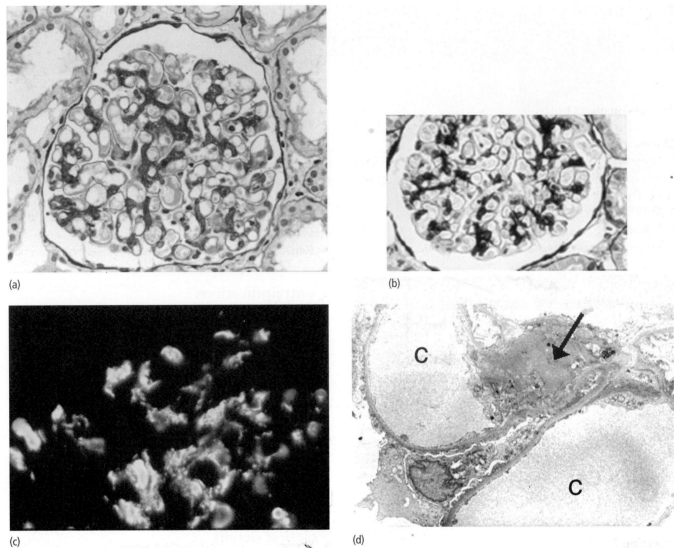

Fig. 112 (a) Light microscopy of a glomerulus. The section has been stained by the periodic acid–Schiff (PAS) method, and shows expansion of the mesangium. (b) Silver-stained section of a glomerulus showing mesangial expansion characteristic of IgA nephropathy. (c) Immunofluorescence for IgA of part of a glomerulus. There is mesangial deposition of IgA. (d) Electron micrograph showing dense deposits in the mesangium, between capillary loops (C). (Courtesy of Dr D Davies, Oxford Radcliffe Hospitals.)

5 When the kidney is reached, the patient is asked to breathe and the needle is seen to swing.
6 The spinal needle is replaced with a biopsy needle, which is passed into the lower pole of the kidney.
7 Usually two cores of tissue are taken.
Special handling of biopsy material is sometimes needed:
- Oxalate nephropathy: alcohol-containing fixative
- Culture for *Mycobacterium tuberculosis*: no fixative.

After the investigation

- Bedrest for 16 h
- Monitor pulse, blood pressure, urine colour.

Complications

The major complication is haemorrhage. Perirenal haematoma is very common (>30%) if looked for by ultrasonography. There is macroscopic haematuria in about 8%. Up to 2% require blood transfusion, and <1% embolization/nephrectomy.

Acknowledgements

The authors are grateful to Drs R.M. Hilton, J.E. Scoble, J.A. Amess and E.C. Morris for their help in sourcing some of the medical images appearing in this book. The editor would also like to thank Dr D. Davies.

4 Self-assessment

Answers on pp. 121–129.

Question 1

A 70-year-old man presented with acute renal failure. No urine was obtained on passing a urinary catheter. Fig. 113 is a CT scan of his abdomen.

1 What is the most obvious abnormality?

2 What are the likely causes?

3 What is the appropriate immediate management?

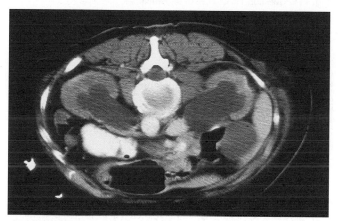

Fig. 113 Question 1.

Question 2

In non-diarrhoeal haemolytic–uraemic syndrome (HUS) (T/F):

A The clotting screen is usually abnormal

B The patient may present with renal failure

C HUS can be precipitated by cyclosporin

D It may be familial

E It is associated with a reduction in von Willebrand factor-cleaving protease.

Question 3

With regard to haemodialysis (T/F):

A Hypotension is made less likely by increasing the target weight

B Fluid removal is mainly controlled by altering the transmembrane pressure

C Osmosis is an important mechanism in the removal of fluid

D High-flux dialysis membranes clear β_2-microglobulin more efficiently

E Convection is the main mechanism of solute removal.

Question 4

Renal transplantation (T/F):

A In the first 6 months after transplantation, mortality is higher than in patients on the transplant waiting list

B Renal transplantation is contraindicated in patients with diabetes

C In the UK, 5 years after transplantation about 40% of grafts will be functioning

D The degree of HLA matching does not influence graft survival

E Renal transplantation is the ideal treatment for renal failure caused by myeloma.

Question 5

Alport's syndrome (T/F):

A Is caused by a defect in the glomerular basement membrane

B Is frequently associated with Goodpasture's disease

C Is usually more severe in girls

D Does not cause significant renal disease in females

E Renal transplantation is contraindicated.

Question 6

Select the single most appropriate answer.

A 76-year-old man has a bladder palpable to the umbilicus. The creatinine is 1000 mol/L and the potassium 8.4 mmol/L. He has Kussmaul's respiration and is drowsy. You would immediately:

A Administer rectal calcium resonium

B Monitor the ECG and inject 10 mL 10% calcium gluconate

C Arrange transfer to a haemodialysis unit

D Infuse 50 mL 50% dextrose with 10 units short-acting insulin

E Arrange transfer to the intensive care unit

F Insert a central venous line

G Infuse 1 litre 1.28% sodium bicarbonate

H Insert a urinary catheter.

Question 7

A 45-year-old man presents with shortness of breath and initial investigations reveal a creatinine of 1200 µmol/L and a haemoglobin of 13.0 g/dL. Shortly after admission to hospital he coughs up some blood and a chest radiograph reveals widespread shadowing.

1 What is the differential diagnosis?

2 What results must be rapidly known?

3 Is it likely that he has acute or chronic renal impairment?

Question 8

For each of the following patients, select the most suitable

113

treatment. Each option may be used once, more than once or not at all.

1 A 36-year-old man with spina bifida and an ileal conduit, who has end-stage renal failure caused by reflux nephropathy and who is wheelchair-bound.

2 A 52-year-old man with acute renal failure following a myocardial infarction complicated by cardiogenic shock.

3 A 76-year-old man with end-stage chronic renal failure who enjoys a very active retirement with frequent walking holidays.

4 An 11-year-old boy nearing end-stage renal failure.

A Home haemodialysis

B Hospital-based haemodialysis

C Live related renal transplant

D Haemofiltration

E Peritoneal dialysis (CAPD)

F Peritoneal dialysis (APD)

G Ultra-low protein diet.

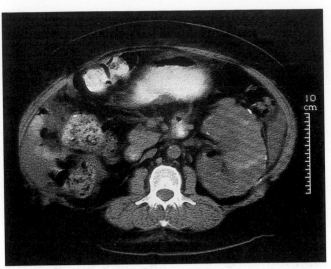

Fig. 114 Question 11: CT scan of abdomen.

Question 9

The following ECG changes commonly occur with severe hyperkalaemia (T/F):

A Prolonged QT interval

B Diminished P wave

C Prominent U wave

D J wave in V5

E Broadened QRS complex.

Question 10

The following may occur after the relief of chronic urinary outflow obstruction (T/F):

A Impaired ability to concentrate urine, which can be improved by administration of antidiuretic hormone (ADH)

B Hypomagnesaemia

C Polyuria

D Hyperkalaemic renal tubular acidosis

E Metabolic acidosis.

Question 11

Fig. 114 is an abdominal CT scan of a haemodialysis patient who has recently had a major operation. Her sister has had a kidney transplant.

1 What is the cause of her renal failure?

2 Can renal transplantation be contemplated in this condition?

3 Give three common presentations of this condition

4 What operation was performed? Give two indications for the operation.

Question 12

Concerning treatment of blood pressure during pregnancy—which of the following statements are true?:

A An ACE inhibitor is the agent of choice for patients with renal impairment and proteinuria after the first trimester

B The threshold for treatment should be higher in the second trimester

C Diuretics are very useful to control oedema

D As a result of its central mode of action, moxonidine is particularly helpful

E α-Methyldopa is usually well tolerated and safe.

Question 13

Estimation of GFR—which of the following statements are true?

A Plasma creatinine normally falls in the second trimester of pregnancy

B Incompletely timed urine collections will over-estimate creatinine clearance

C The GFR of each surviving nephron is reduced in chronic renal failure

D Trimethoprim reduces creatinine clearance

E Decreasing protein intake reduces creatinine clearance.

Question 14

Presentation in renal disease—for each of the following scenarios, select the most likely underlying diagnosis. Each option may be used once, more than once or not at all.

A 28-year-old woman with proteinuria, renal impairment and history of childhood urinary tract infection

B 40-year-old woman with hypertension and an episode of haematuria whose mother died of renal failure aged 60

C 21-year-old man with repeated episodes of macroscopic haematuria

D 68-year-old woman with hypercalcaemia, renal impairment and history of renal stones

E 46-year-old man found at insurance medical to have hypertension and microscopic haematuria.

1 Autosomal dominant polycystic kidney disease

2 Alport's syndrome

3 Goodpasture's syndrome (antiglomerular basement membrane antibodies)

4 IgA nephropathy

5 Reflux nephropathy

6 Primary hyperparathyroidism

7 Multiple myeloma.

Question 15

Interpretation of skull radiograph. Fig. 115 shows a plain radiograph of the skull. Select the statements you consider to be correct:

A The patient has evidence of multiple myeloma

B The patient has hyperparathyroidism

C The patient has evidence of a pituitary tumour

D The appearances are normal.

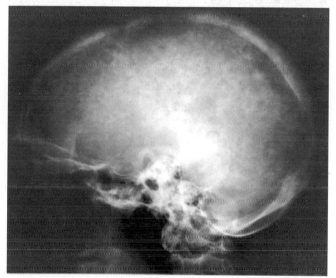

Fig. 115 Question 15: skull radiograph.

Question 16

Interpretation of 24-h collection: calculate the creatinine clearance from the following information about a 35-year-old man. Comment on the value obtained.

Plasma creatinine: 124 µmol/L

Patient's weight: 76 kg

24-h urine volume: 1.2 L

Urine creatinine concentration: 5.1 mmol/L.

Question 17

Parathyroid function—which of the following statements are true?

A In normal individuals, hypophosphataemia stimulates production of PTH

B Aluminium hydroxide is the preferred phosphate binder in dialysis patients

C There are normally five parathyroid glands

D Inactivation of parathyroid hormone is mainly achieved through removal by glomerular filtration

E Parathyroid carcinoma is a frequent complication of prolonged renal replacement therapy.

Question 18

Erythropoietin and renal anaemia—which of the following statements are true?

A Treatment with erythropoietin is not permitted by Muslims

B Patients with polycystic kidney disease tend to need increased doses of erythropoietin

C Erythropoietin should be administered intravenously

D Intercurrent infections reduce responsiveness to erythropoietin

E Antibodies to erythropoietin are a common clinical problem.

Question 19

Renin—which of the following statements are true?

A Renin levels tend to be higher when ambulant than when recumbent

B Renin levels are elevated after bilateral nephrectomy

C Renin is produced by the proximal tubule mitochondria

D ACE inhibitors lower renin levels

E Renin is characteristically low in patients with Conn's syndrome.

Question 20

Nephrotic syndrome: at renal biopsy, the following pathological diagnoses have been made in 45-year-old women presenting with nephrotic syndrome and normal creatinine clearance. Weight is 60 kg. Select the most appropriate statement concerning the initial therapeutic strategy in each case. Each option may be used once, more than once or not at all.

A Membranous glomerulonephritis

B Minimal change nephrotic syndrome

C Focal segmental glomerulosclerosis

D Primary amyloid.

1 Oral prednisolone 60 mg/day

2 Symptomatic treatment of oedema, control hypertension, monitor GFR

3 Consider chemotherapy with stem-cell transplantation

4 Oral prednisolone 15 mg/day.

Question 21

Peritoneal dialysis (T/F):

A Usually results in 5 g or more loss of albumin per day in the dialysate

B Allows unrestricted intake of dietary phosphate in most patients

C Is especially suitable for obese patients

D Fluid removal relies on osmosis

E Should be avoided in patients with autosomal dominant polycystic kidney disease.

Question 22

Diet in renal disease: for each food, select the component that is most likely to lead to restricted intake in patients treated by dialysis. Each option may be used once, more than once or not at all.

A Milk

115

B Oranges
C Instant coffee
D Tomatoes
E Cheese
F Bacon
G Baked potatoes.
1 Potassium
2 Phosphate
3 Sodium
4 Magnesium.

Question 23

Drug and toxin exposure and the kidney: for each toxin/drug, select one statement concerning its effect on the renal tract. Each option may be used once, more than once or not at all.
A Cyclophosphamide
B Gold
C Mercury
D Ampicillin
E Penicillamine
F Acyclovir
G Lead.
1 Haemorrhagic cystitis
2 Acute interstitial nephritis
3 Membranous nephropathy
4 Focal segmental glomerulonephritis
5 Chronic interstitial nephritis
6 Obstructive uropathy caused by crystalluria.

Question 24

Immunofluorescence in renal biopsies: for each diagnosis select the expected findings in the glomerulus on immunofluorescence.
A SLE
B Goodpasture's syndrome
C Henoch–Schönlein purpura
D ANCA-positive vasculitis
E Acute tubular necrosis
F Membranous glomerulonephritis.
1 Linear deposition of IgG
2 Minimal deposition of immunoglobulins
3 Mesangial IgA deposition
4 Granular deposition of IgG
5 Deposition of IgG, IgA, IgM and complement.

Question 25

A 70-year-old man with extensive non-Hodgkin's lymphoma is treated with chemotherapy; 36 h later he is oligoanuric (Table 26).
1 What do you consider the most likely diagnosis and how would you confirm it?
2 How would you treat the patient?
3 If contacted before the chemotherapy, what would you have suggested?

Table 26 Question 25.

	Admission	Time of referral
Creatinine (mol/L)	93	302
Potassium (mmol/L)	4.6	7.2
Calcium (mmol/L)	2.3	1.9
Phosphate (mmol/L)	1.2	2.6
Bicarbonate (mmol/L)	26	15

Question 26

Which of the following statements are true of diabetic nephropathy?
A It is the underlying renal diagnosis in over 20% of dialysis patients in the UK
B There is a higher mortality than in patients with other forms of nephropathy
C Microalbuminuria occurs in over 50% of patients with type I diabetes over the course of their disease
D Kimmelstiel–Wilson nodules are the most usual abnormality on renal histology
E Blood pressure control can usually be achieved with an angiotensin-converting enzyme inhibitor alone.

Question 27

Fig. 116 shows an electron micrograph of part of a glomerulus. Identify the structures indicated. Comment on the appearance of the glomerulus.

Question 28

In analgesic nephropathy (T/F):
A There is often salt wasting
B The IVU appearances are distinguishable from reflux nephropathy
C Nephrocalcinosis may be present

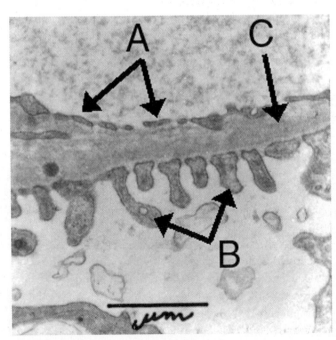

Fig. 116 Question 27. (Courtesy of Dr D Davies.)

D There may be macroscopic haematuria
E Renal biopsy is usually performed to establish the diagnosis.

Question 29

In patients with renal failure associated with multiple myeloma, which of the following statements are true?
A Hypercalcaemia rarely contributes to ARF
B Intratubular casts are typical
C Recovery from renal failure should be anticipated in most cases
D A 1-year survival rate of about 50% is expected when dialysis becomes necessary
E With ARF, chemotherapy for the myeloma should be withheld until the ARF resolves.

Question 30

Which of the following are true of renal tubular acidosis (RTA)?
A Renal stone formation is seen only in RTA-2
B Hypokalaemia occurs in all types of RTA
C RTA-1 and RTA-2 may both complicate Sjögren's syndrome
D Patients with RTA-1 can never acidify their urine
E Oral bicarbonate replacement is greater in RTA-2 than in RTA-1.

Question 31

For each of the following conditions, select the most appropriate investigation for determining the diagnosis from the options above. Each option may be used once, more than once or not at all.
A Focal segmental glomerulosclerosis
B Renal artery stenosis
C Adult polycystic kidney disease
D Interstitial nephritis.
1 Ultrasonography
2 Renal biopsy
3 Midstream urine microscopy and culture
4 Renal angiography
5 Peripheral blood count
6 Bone marrow examination.

Question 32

A young man presents with a sudden onset of severe colicky loin pain. Dipstick analysis reveals microscopic haematuria +++. Which is the most likely diagnosis?
A Minimal change nephropathy
B Renal artery stenosis
C Acute tubular necrosis
D Urinary stone disease
E IgA nephropathy.

Question 33

A previously well 75-year-old man attending his general practitioner for a routine health check is found to have a plasma creatinine of 240 µmol/L. On reviewing the notes, it appeared that his creatinine was 140 µmol/L 2 years previously. He is on no medication.
1 What are the likely causes of his renal impairment?
2 What specific questions would you ask him?
3 What investigations may be diagnostically useful?

Question 34

An elderly man who smokes is admitted for femoropopliteal bypass surgery for symptomatic peripheral vascular disease. He has a strong family history of vascular disease and is hyperlipidaemic. His blood pressure is 190/100. He is otherwise well, but baseline investigations reveal a plasma creatinine of 250 µmol/L.
The most likely diagnosis is:
A Interstitial nephritis
B Alport's disease
C Minimal change nephropathy
D Renal artery stenosis
E Rapidly progressive glomerulonephritis.

Question 35

Fig. 117 shows a renal biopsy from a 55-year-old man with a rash, eosinophilia and acute renal failure.
1 What is the diagnosis?
2 Give two events that could have precipitated this illness.

Question 36

For each of the conditions listed below, select the most likely typical causative pathogen. Each option may be used once, more than once or not at all.
1 Renal amyloidosis
2 Haemolytic–uraemic syndrome
3 Membranous nephropathy
4 Focal segmental glomerulosclerosis.
A Hepatitis C
B Hepatitis B
C Group A streptococci

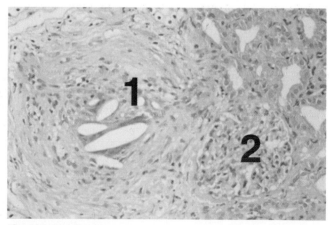

Fig. 117 Question 35.

D *Escherichia coli* strain 0157
E *Mycobacterium tuberculosis*
F *Proteus mirabilis*
G Human immunodeficiency virus.

Question 37

Which of the following renal conditions are typically seen in systemic lupus erythematosus?
A Minimal change nephropathy
B Focal segmental glomerulosclerosis
C Diffuse proliferative glomerulonephritis
D Membranous glomerulonephritis
E Renal artery stenosis.

Question 38

For each of the conditions listed below, select the most likely associated haematological abnormality. Each option may be used once, more than once or not at all.
1 Systemic lupus erythematosus
2 Myeloma
3 Acute interstitial nephritis
4 Haemolytic–uraemic syndrome.
A Microangiopathic haemolytic anaemia
B Rouleaux
C Eosinophilia
D Lymphocytopenia
E A shortened kaolin-cephalin clotting time (KCCT)
F Megaloblastic anaemia
G Nucleated red blood cells.

Question 39

A 38-year-old intravenous heroin user presents with a history of swollen ankles. Urinalysis reveals heavy proteinuria and his plasma creatinine is 256 µmol/L and his plasma albumin 21 g/L.
1 What are the possible diagnoses?
2 What investigations are necessary?
3 What advice would you give the patient?

Question 40

Which of the following types of renal stones are visible on a plain radiograph?:
A Cystine stones
B Uric acid stones
C Infection stones
D Calcium oxalate stones
E Xanthine stones.

Question 41

A 28-year-old woman presents with general malaise. On examination, she is found to have an early diastolic murmur at the lower left sternal edge. This was not noted on an insurance medical only 3 months previously. On dipstick analysis, there is haematuria+ and proteinuria+. Her creat-inine is 230 µmol/L. Her creatinine had been only 80 µmol/L when she had the insurance medical.
1 What are the two most likely diagnoses?
2 How would you investigate this woman further?

Question 42

For each of the systemic diseases listed below, select the most likely associated renal tract pathology. Each option may be used once, more than once or not at all.
1 Diabetes mellitus
2 Hypertension
3 Systemic vasculitis
4 Schistosomiasis.
A Membranous nephropathy
B Bladder carcinoma
C Glomerular sclerosis
D Crescentic glomerulonephritris
E Membranous nephropathy
F Retroperitonal fibrosis
G Pelviureteric junction obstruction.

Question 43

A 21-year-old woman is referred with a creatinine of 221 µmol/L. Her mother attends with her and reports that, as a small baby, she had repeated urine infections which made her unwell. Her renal function has been checked every year since she was very young and has been slowly deteriorating. She has not had symptomatic urinary tract infections for years, but is now pregnant.
1 What is the likely diagnosis?
2 Is it relevant that she is now pregnant?
3 What are the implications for her baby?

Question 44

Fig. 118 shows two renal biopsies from patients with acute renal failure. For each, select the most appropriate statement.
1 The biopsy shows a crescentic glomerulonephritis
2 The patient is likely to have myeloma
3 The biopsy shows acute tubular necrosis
4 The biopsy shows intimal proliferation in a blood vessel
5 The biopsy shows a granulomatous interstitial nephritis.

Question 45

Which of the following statements concerning renal biopsy findings are true?
A A focal glomerulonephritis refers to a process affecting some, but not all, glomeruli
B A segmental glomerulonephritis refers to a process affecting some, but not all, glomeruli
C Crescents on a renal biopsy indicate a slow and non-aggressive disease process
D Interstitial nephritis refers to inflammation affecting the blood vessel walls
E Acute tubular necrosis can be diagnosed on a renal biopsy.

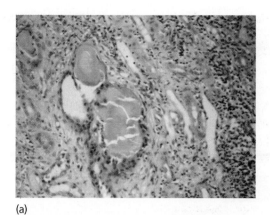

(a)

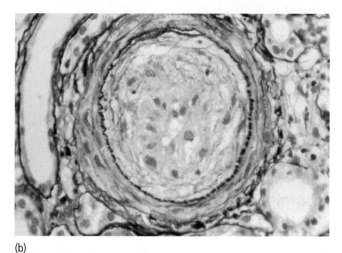

(b)

Fig. 118 Question 44.

Question 46

In a patient with acute renal colic, which of the following statements are true?

A A typical site for stones to lodge is where the ureter enters the bladder

B Proteinuria is a typical finding

C There is invariably a dramatic rise in plasma creatinine

D The patient should avoid fluids as these worsen the pain

E Pain may be referred to the tip of the scapula.

Question 47

For each of the clinical scenarios listed below, select the most likely associated renal condition. Each option may be used once, more than once or not at all.

1 A young man with recurrent frank haematuria occurring with upper respiratory tract infections

2 An 11-year-old boy with a 2-day history of swollen ankles and frothy urine

3 An elderly man with a known malignancy, renal impairment and nephrotic syndrome

4 An acute fall in urine volume and haemoptysis.

A Rhabdomyolysis

B Goodpasture's s disease

C IgA nephropathy

D Systemic lupus erythematosus

E Mesangiocapillary glomerulonephritis

F Minimal change nephropathy

G Membranous nephropathy.

Question 48

Which of the following statements concerning urinary tract infection are true?

A Tuberculosis does not affect the urinary tract

B Adult polycystic kidney disease is a risk factor

C Upper urinary tract infection is increased in pregnancy

D *Staphylococcus aureus* is a common cause

E *Candida albicans* is a common cause.

Question 49

For each of the renal diseases listed below, select the most likely associated serological finding. Each option may be used once, more than once or not at all.

1 Mesangiocapillary glomerulonephritis associated with hepatitis C virus infection

2 IgA nephropathy

3 Membranous nephropathy associated with systemic lupus erythematosus

4 Crescentic glomerulonephritis associated with Wegener's granulomatosis.

A A high titre of ANCA (antineutrophil cytoplasmic antibody).

B Antibodies against double-stranded DNA

C A raised plasma IgA level

D Antimitochondrial antibodies

E Cryoglobulins

F Cold agglutinins

G A raised antistreptolysin O titre.

Question 50

Which of the following are true?

A Life expectancy of non-diabetic patients under 40 years of age treated with haemodialysis is similar to an age-matched population without renal disease

B Carpal tunnel syndrome in dialysis patients is usually the result of oedema

C Plasma homocyst(e)ine levels are elevated in dialysis patients

D Cholecalciferol has advantages over other vitamin D analogues in preventing renal bone disease

E Haemodialysis patients treated with erythropoietin are prone to iron overload.

Question 51

Which of the following lead to the elimination of potassium from the body?

A Intravenous dextrose and insulin

B Intravenous insulin

C Intravenous calcium gluconate

D Rectal administration of 30 g calcium resonium ion exchange resin

E Nebulized salbutamol.

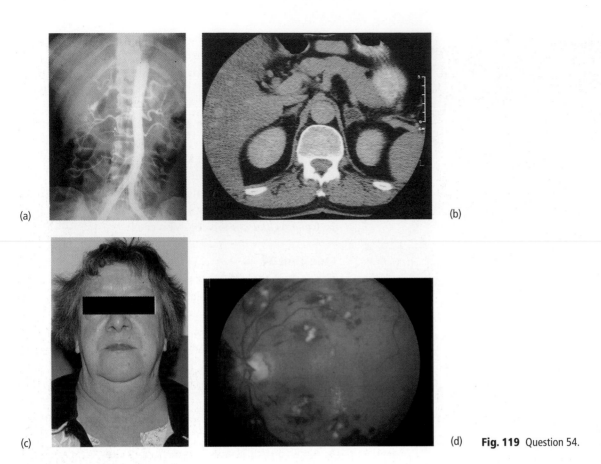

(a)

(b)

(c)

(d) **Fig. 119** Question 54.

Question 52

Select the most likely cause of ARF for each clinical situation. Each option may be used once, more than once or not at all.

1 A 58-year-old man undergoes coronary angiography. One week later he is admitted with ARF and mottling of the skin of his toes.

2 A 22-week pregnant woman, known to have a solitary hypertrophied kidney, is admitted with a fever, loin tenderness and ARF.

3 A patient undergoes large bowel resection for malignancy, but 4 days later is noticed to have a faecal leak from the abdominal wound. She has an abdominal CT scan with contrast, which demonstrates the anastomotic dehiscence; 24 h later she is oliguric.

A Crescentic glomerulonephritis
B Radiocontrast nephropathy
C Cholesterol atheroemboli
D Acute tubular necrosis
E Acute pyelonephritis
F Rhabdomyolysis
G Haemolytic–uraemic syndrome.

Question 53

For each of the following drugs, select the most appropriate statement concerning their use in people with diabetes who have renal impairment:

1 Insulin
2 Glibenclamide
3 Lisinopril
4 Suxamethonium
5 Co-proxamol
6 Metformin
7 Simvastatin
8 Alfacalcidol.
A Reduced elimination and prolonged action
B May exacerbate hyperkalaemia
C Accumulation of active metabolites
D Risk of lactic acidosis
E May cause hypercalcaemia
F No contraindication.

Question 54

Fig. 119 shows investigations/appearances from four different patients. Three have secondary hypertension. For each, describe the abnormality and indicate which patient does not have hypertension.

Question 55

Explain whether you would prescribe a non-steroidal anti-inflammatory drug for joint pains in a woman with renal impairment and a multi-system disease.

Answers to Self-assessment

Answer to Question 1

1 This CT scan shows gross bilateral hydronephrosis. The empty bladder suggests bilateral upper tract obstruction.
2 The most common cause is malignancy; in particular, prostate cancer can spread to encase the ureters. Also consider retroperitoneal fibrosis.
3 The immediate management is to relieve the obstruction with nephrostomies or by retrograde insertion of stents (see Section 2.6, p. 88).

Answer to Question 2

F, T, T, T, F

An abnormal clotting screen should suggest another diagnosis such as sepsis with disseminated vascular coagulation (DIC). Renal failure is a common presenting feature of HUS. Cyclosporin is a recognized cause. There are a number of familial reports of HUS. Some have been associated with deficiency of factor H, a plasma protein involved in regulating the alternative pathway of complement activation. Thrombotic, thrombocytopenic purpura (TTP) has been linked to reduced von Willebrand factor-cleaving protease activity.

Answer to Question 3

T, T, F, T, F

Hypotension commonly occurs during haemodialysis. Important factors are the rate of fluid removal and the final volume status. Ultrafiltration is mainly achieved by a pressure gradient, not osmosis. High flux membranes have bigger pores that allow better clearance of middle molecules such as β_2-microglobulin. There is some solute transport associated with ultrafiltration through convection, but diffusion is the main mechanism involved in toxin removal (see Section 2.2, p. 61).

Answer to Question 4

T, F, F, F, F

The mortality after transplantation is initially higher than for patients remaining on the waiting list; however, after 1 year survival is superior to those remaining on dialysis. Transplantation in patients with diabetes is particularly beneficial in terms of mortality. HLA matching does affect outcome and 5-year graft survival rate is between 65% and 75%. Transplanting patients with myeloma, even if apparently disease free, can be hazardous with a high recurrence and death rate (see Section 2.2, p. 69).

Answer to Question 5

T, F, F, F, F

Alport's syndrome is usually caused by a mutation in the *COL4A5* gene. The gene is on the X chromosome, and female carriers are usually much less severely affected than males, although they frequently have microscopic haematuria and may have renal impairment. The autoantigen in Goodpasture's disease is absent in Alport's syndrome (see Section 2.8.2, p. 104).

Answer to Question 6

B

The danger is of cardiac dysrhythmia related to hyperkalaemia. The most rapid cardioprotection will be provided by intravenous calcium. Subsequent manoeuvres will include D and G. Monitoring on the intensive care unit may be appropriate if a bed is available, but should not delay therapy. Transfer to a haemodialysis unit will be unnecessary if there is a good diuresis after insertion of a urinary catheter. Rectal calcium resonium is unpleasant and not indicated here!

Answer to Question 7

1 The man has renal failure and haemoptysis with widespread pulmonary changes on a radiograph. This pulmonary disease could be diffuse alveolar haemorrhage. However, it could also be pulmonary oedema with rupture of a dilated vessel causing some haemoptysis. Alternatively, it could represent infection. These possibilities could all be associated with renal disease. Goodpasture's disease can cause renal failure and diffuse alveolar haemorrhage. Renal failure can itself contribute to pulmonary oedema as a result of inadequate renal capacity for water excretion and consequent volume overload. Sepsis, if serious, can be associated with acute renal failure.
2 In any patient suddenly discovered to have severe renal impairment, it is essential to know whether the patient's potassium level is dangerously high. This is especially so in acute renal failure where compensatory changes across the plasma membrane will have had less time to occur. It is also important to check the arterial blood gases to ensure that the patient is not dangerously acidotic or hypoxic. If there is severe hyperkalaemia, acidosis or dangerous pulmonary oedema, then, in the absence of renal function, the patient must be haemofiltered or haemodialysed.
3 The normal haemoglobin suggests that this is acute renal failure, although in the absence of other information it is difficult to be sure.

Answer to Question 8

1B, 2D, 3E, 4C
See Sections 1.5 and 2.2 (pp. 13–15 and 61–72).

Answer to Question 9

F, T, F, F, T

Prolonged QT interval and prominent U waves are seen in congenital syndromes (Romano–Ward), secondary to antiarrhythmic drugs (sotalol, amiodarone, quinidine), and in hypocalcaemia, hypokalaemia and hypomagnesaemia. J waves are associated with hypothermia.

Answer to Question 10
T, T, T, T, T
Tubular dysfunction is often marked in this setting, and can lead to all these abnormalities.

Answer to Question 11
1 This scan demonstrates a single enlarged irregular multicystic kidney. The diagnosis is polycystic kidney disease.
2 Transplantation is not contraindicated, but in some patients the kidneys are sufficiently large to make transplantation difficult.
3 Other presentations include hypertension, haematuria, abdominal pain, urinary tract infection and (rarely) subarachnoid haemorrhage.
4 The operation was a nephrectomy, which may be indicated for chronic pain, bleeding, recurrent infection or to make space for a transplant (see Section 2.8, pp. 102–103).

Answer to Question 12
F, F, F, F, T
There is clear evidence that ACE inhibitors in the second and third trimester can have serious adverse effects on the fetus. A very restricted range of drugs, including α-methyldopa, and hydralazine have been shown to be safe in pregnancy. Newer agents such as moxonidine are unlikely to be tested or licensed for use in pregnancy. The blood pressure normally falls in the second trimester, so the threshold for concern and treatment is lower.

Answer to Question 13
T, F, F, T, T
Creatinine falls in the second trimester as the GFR increases. Incomplete collections will under-estimate creatinine excretion and hence creatinine clearance. Individual surviving nephrons increase their filtration rate as the total GFR falls. Trimethoprim reduces tubular secretion of creatinine, decreasing creatinine clearance without altering GFR. The GFR can increase by up to 20% with protein loading.

Answer to Question 14
A5, B1, C4, D6, E4

Answer to Question 15
D
The radiograph shows the classic 'pepperpot' appearances of hyperparathyroidism.

Answer to Question 16
Creatine clearance = urine creatinine concentration (μmol/L) × urine production (mL/min) concentration in plasma (μmol/L)

$$5100 \times (1200/(24 \times 60))/124 = 34.3 \text{ mL/min}$$

Comments: this is a low value for a man of this age; it is lower than expected given the plasma creatinine; 24-h collection is almost certainly incomplete, because creatinine excretion is expected to be 12 mmol if lean body weight is 70 kg.

Answer to Question 17
F, F, F, F, F
Hypophosphataemia tends to suppress PTH secretion. Aluminium compounds are avoided if possible, although they are effective since aluminium accumulation is a major risk. There are normally four parathyroid glands. Inactivation of PTH is mainly by cleavage in the liver. Parathyroid carcinoma is very rare indeed (approximately 100 cases in the world literature).

Answer to Question 18
F, F, F, T, F
Erythropoietin that is used clinically is produced from hamster tissue culture cells transfected with the human erythropoietin gene. Polycystic patients have relatively preserved erythropoietin production, and often do not need exogenous erythropoietin. Although effective intravenously, subcutaneous administration is more cost-effective. Any acute phase response decreases the response to erythropoietin. Antierythropoietin antibodies in patients treated with the two available preparations of recombinant human erythropoietin have not been documented.

Answer to Question 19
T, F, F, F, T
Renin secretion is stimulated in the erect position, and is produced by the granular cells of the juxtaglomerular apparatus, which are modified smooth muscle cells in the afferent arteriole. ACE inhibitors result in a marked stimulation of renin secretion. In primary hyperaldosteronism renin is suppressed.

Answer to Question 20
A2, B1, C1, D3
Over 90% of adults with minimal change nephrotic syndrome will respond to prednisolone 1 mg/kg, although response frequently takes longer than in children. Randomized trials suggest that steroids alone are not beneficial in membranous nephropathy, and a significant number of patients (about 30%) will undergo a spontaneous complete or partial remission. Immunosuppressive regimens are usually reserved for those with deteriorating renal function over a period of 6–12 months. Focal segmental glomerulosclerosis responds to steroids (1 mg/kg), with a complete or partial remission in up to 60% of adults. The long-term outlook for renal function is much better in responders than in non-responders. Remission often takes longer than in minimal change nephrotic syndrome. Primary

amyloid is caused by an autonomous B-cell clone. The outlook of patients with renal disease alone is relatively good, but the only potentially curative treatment is eradication of the B-cell clone.

Answer to Question 21
T, F, F, T, F

Peritoneal dialysis usually leads to the loss of large amounts of albumin in the dialysate. Phosphate restriction and phosphate binders are almost always required in dialysis patients. Glucose is absorbed from the dialysate, so weight gain is a common problem. Fluid removal is achieved by osmosis using hypertonic dialysate (see Section 2.2, p. 65).

Answer to Question 22
A2, B1, C1, D1, E2, F3, G1

• Potassium: instant coffee, fruit and chocolate are all high in potassium. Potatoes should be boiled with skin removed.
• Phosphate: all proteins contain phosphate, so effective restriction is difficult. Dairy foods are particularly high in phosphate and intake is usually restricted.
• Sodium: sodium intake is important for blood pressure and fluid control. Salt should usually be avoided in cooking and not added. Salty foods, which include many processed foods, also need to be avoided.
• Magnesium tends to be a problem only when it is being taken in medicines (e.g. antacids and laxatives).

Answer to Question 23
A1, B3, C3, D2, E3, F6, G5

Answer to Question 24
A5, B1, C3, D2, E2, F4

In SLE nephritis, a wide range of different histological features is seen. There is usually marked immunoglobulin and complement deposition. Goodpasture's syndrome is caused by antibody to the GBM, visible as linear deposition of IgG. Henoch–Schönlein purpura is associated with mesangial IgA deposition, forming part of the spectrum of IgA nephropathy. ANCA-positive vasculitis is also described as pauci-immune because of the lack of immunoglobulin deposition. Acute tubular necrosis is not associated with deposition of complement in the glomerulus.

Answer to Question 25
1 The clinical setting and laboratory findings are typical of tumour lysis syndrome. Plasma urate is likely to be very high (>900 µmol/L). Renal failure is caused by urate crystals in the tubules.
2 Commence allopurinol (decreases urate production). Administer intravenous fluids and a loop diuretic to establish a diuresis. If this fails to institute a brisk diuresis, treat with haemodialysis which is very efficient at removing uric acid from the circulation.

3 Commence allopurinol. This is a competitive antagonist of xanthine oxidase, so a higher dose than normal is used (600 or 900 mg/day). Diuresis of at least 2.5 L per day is recommended. Usually intravenous fluids will be needed to achieve this.

Answer to Question 26
T, T, T, F, F

The greatly increased relative risk of death in patients with diabetic nephropathy is the result of cardiovascular disease. Patients with diabetes account for over 20% of patients on dialysis programmes and this figure may be greater in areas of higher ethnicity, where diabetic prevalence is increased. Kimmelstiel–Wilson lesions (nodular sclerosis) are considered specific for diabetic nephropathy, but diffuse mesangial thickening and sclerosis are the most common histological changes seen on renal biopsy. Multiple antihypertensive agents are usually required to obtain blood pressure control in diabetic nephropathy.

Answer to Question 27
A Endothelium (fenestrated).
B Epithelial foot processes
C Glomerular basement membrane
Comment: the appearances are those of a normal peripheral capillary loop.

Answer to Question 28
T, T, T, T, F

In analgesic nephropathy, the typical cup and spill deformities of papillary necrosis can be seen on IVU; the papillae may calcify. The condition predisposes to the development of urothelial malignancy. The diagnosis can be established if the characteristic IVU findings are accompanied by a history of analgesic abuse.

Answer to Question 29
F, T, F, T, F

Myeloma commonly involves the kidney and typical histological features include fractured intratubular casts, tubular atrophy and multi-nucleate giant cells. ARF develops in 7% of patients with myeloma, and a higher proportion develop progressive renal failure; renal recovery is the exception rather than the rule. In those patients who develop end-stage renal failure, a 1-year survival rate of 50% may be expected.

Answer to Question 30
F, F, T, T, T

Distal RTA (type 1) is characterized by nephrocalcinosis and urinary stone formation. The primary defect is failure to acidify urine, and the quantities of bicarbonate required to treat the acidosis are far less than in RTA-2, in which proximal tubular bicarbonate wasting occurs. In RTA-1 the urine pH is always >5.4, but patients with RTA-2 may be able to acidify their urine (as a result of a threshold effect for bicarbonate reabsorption). Hyperkalaemia occurs in RTA-4 and is related to aldosterone deficiency.

Answer to Question 31

A2, B4, C1, D2

For any glomerular disease, the diagnosis is usually made by renal biopsy. Although other investigations often indicate a likely diagnosis, a renal biopsy is usually necessary. This is also the case for interstitial nephritis. Renal artery stenosis is difficult to exclude unless angiography has been performed, and sampling of renal vein renin levels has not proved useful in clinical practice. Adult polycystic kidney disease can, in some families, be diagnosed by genetic means. However, the mutations vary from family to family and spontaneous new mutations in unaffected families are well recognized. For this reason, imaging remains the mainstay of diagnosis.

Answer to Question 32

D

Although pain can occur with acute glomerulonephritis, this is certainly uncommon and is not a feature of minimal change nephropathy. Colicky pain typically occurs in urinary obstruction, usually caused by a ureteric stone; this is consistent with the microscopic haematuria. IgA nephropathy certainly causes haematuria and sometimes, when there is macroscopic haematuria, it is associated with loin pain, although the history and findings here are more consistent with a stone. Renal artery stenosis does not usually cause either pain or haematuria. Colicky pain is not a feature of acute tubular necrosis.

Answer to Question 33

1 In any older man, it is essential to remember that both benign and malignant prostatic disease can cause postrenal obstruction and renal impairment. In addition, hypertension and diabetes mellitus are both common in elderly people and can both cause renal impairment. Renal artery stenosis is also a possible cause of renal impairment. Obviously, chronic glomerulonephritis can occur in elderly people as can renal disease associated with myeloma.

2 It is important to ask specifically about symptoms relating to prostatic disease. Is his urinary stream good? Does he have hesitancy, terminal dribbling or excessive frequency or nocturia or incontinence? It is essential to check for a palpable bladder and to perform a rectal examination to assess the prostate.

3 Basic investigations must include ultrasonography which may show obstruction. Urinalysis and microscopy will narrow the differential diagnosis. In addition, it is wise to check the prostate-specific antigen if there is any indication of prostatic disease. In elderly men with renal impairment, plasma and urine electrophoresis should be performed because myeloma and amyloid are relatively common. Other investigations that may be performed depending on these results include renal biopsy and renal angiography.

Answer to Question 34

D

Minimal change nephropathy does not normally cause renal impairment. Although the other conditions can all cause renal impairment, the most likely diagnosis in a man with known vascular disease, hypertension and renal impairment is renal artery stenosis.

Answer to Question 35

Cholesterol emboli. The biopsy shows clefts where cholesterol crystals have dissolved in processing (labelled 1) The glomerulus (labelled 2) is normal. Cholesterol embolization is usually precipitated by angiography (e.g. coronary or renal) or less commonly by thrombolysis.

Answer to Question 36

1E, 2D, 3B, 4G

All the organisms listed can cause renal or urinary tract disease. Hepatitis C is associated with mesangiocapillary glomerulonephritis. Group A streptococci are the causative organisms in the diffuse proliferative glomerulonephritis of poststreptococcal disease. *Proteus* species are often responsible for urinary tract infection, especially in the presence of urinary tract stones.

Answer to Question 37

T, F, T, T, F

Systemic lupus erythematosus can cause a range of renal pathological appearances. The best recognized are those encapsulated by the classification of the National Institutes of Health (NIH). These are: minimal change nephropathy, mesangial glomerulonephritis, focal proliferative glomerulonephritis, diffuse proliferative glomerulonephritis (± crescents) and membranous nephropathy. There is also often a tubular or an interstitial component to the renal disease.

Answer to Question 38

1D, 2B, 3C, 4A

Systemic lupus erythematosus can cause anaemia, thrombocytopenia and general leucocytopenia (a low total white cell count), which is usually most characterized by lymphopenia (a low lymphocyte count). In the presence of a so-called lupus anticoagulant, the KCCT is typically prolonged in lupus. Acute interstitial nephritis can be associated with both eosinophilia and eosinophiluria.

Answer to Question 39

1 It is likely that the patient has nephrotic syndrome as a result of an underlying glomerulonephritis. In black intravenous heroin users, a focal segmental glomerulosclerosis has been associated with HIV infection and this is certainly a possible diagnosis. However, any other cause of renal impairment and nephrotic syndrome such as membranous nephropathy or amyloidosis is possible. AA amyloidosis is worth considering in a patient who may be at risk of tuberculosis. Intravenous drug addicts are also at risk of infection with hepatitis viruses; hepatitis B virus is associated with membranous nephropathy and hepatitis C virus with mesangiocapillary glomerulonephritis.

2 A renal biopsy will be necessary to make the renal diagnosis, and serology should be checked for the relevant viral infections. Any other potential infections, such as TB, should be sought if there are relevant clinical pointers.

3 The advice given to the patient will depend on the findings. Clearly, it would be better if they could stop using intravenous drugs. If they are infected with a serious virus, then any available treatment for that will be indicated. In addition, the patient must be advised about his or her infectivity with respect to other people, and particularly about the use of shared needles for intravenous drug administration.

Answer to Question 40

T, F, T, T, F

All calcium-containing stones are radio-opaque and infection stones contain calcium. Cystine stones are also, to a lesser extent, radio-opaque. However, xanthine and uric acid stones are radiolucent and are not visible on plain radiography. If appropriate views can be obtained, all stone types can be detected by ultrasonography.

Answer to Question 41

1 The most likely diagnoses in the presence of a new murmur and renal impairment are infective endocarditis and SLE. The murmur is that of aortic regurgitation. It is critical to distinguish the two because the treatment for lupus would be immunosuppression and this could be catastrophic if given to a patient with infective endocarditis. Both lupus and infective endocarditis are associated with glomerulonephritis.

2 It is essential to exclude infective endocarditis, by repeated blood cultures and transthoracic and often transoesophageal echocardiography. Typically, in lupus the ESR is high and the CRP is low, whereas, in infective endocarditis, both the CRP and ESR may be elevated. Both lupus and infective endocarditis can cause low complement levels. Autoantibodies can arise during infective endocarditis, but antibodies to double-stranded DNA are highly suggestive of lupus. Ultimately, a renal biopsy may be necessary, although it may not clearly distinguish the two conditions.

Answer to Question 42

1C, 2C, 3D, 4B

Both diabetes and hypertension can cause glomerular sclerosis or scarring. Systemic vasculitis is an important cause of crescentic glomerulonephritis. Some forms of schistosomiasis cause chronic infection of the urinary tract and granulomatous disease, which can ultimately result in bladder cancer.

Answer to Question 43

1 The likely diagnosis is that she had vesicoureteric reflux as a small child. This would have predisposed her to upper urinary tract infection at an early age and these recurrent infections could have caused substantial renal damage. Over the years, her renal function has slowly deteriorated as a result.

2 The reflux itself often resolves, but the renal damage is permanent. She now has chronic renal impairment. Chronic renal impairment of any cause can worsen during pregnancy and may also make the pregnancy less optimal, with an increased risk of complications. However, she does have a progressive chronic renal failure and, over time, her fertility will be reduced. For this reason, the patient may wish to risk the further renal damage that the pregnancy may cause in order to start her family while she can still do so. However, all this requires careful discussion with the patient.

3 There is evidence that vesicoureteric reflux is more common in the children of affected mothers. As most of the damage occurs at an early age, it is now wise to screen such babies so that they can be monitored or treated prophylactically to avoid renal damage. Screening usually consists of a micturating cystoureterogram to look for reflux. The reflux itself usually resolves as the child grows, so the priority is simply to avoid renal damage from upper urinary tract infection.

Answer to Question 44

(a) 2—the biopsy shows a 'fractured' cast with interstitial inflammation. The patient was found to have a paraprotein.

(b) 4—there is marked intimal proliferation in an arteriole. This patient with scleroderma had a classic renal crisis with hypertension and renal failure (see Section 2.3, p. 72).

Answer to Question 45

T, F, F, F, T

A focal glomerulonephritis affects some but not all glomeruli, whereas a diffuse glomerulonephritis affects all the glomeruli. A segmental glomerulonephritis affects only a portion within the affected glomeruli, whereas a global glomerulonephritis affects all portions of affected glomeruli. Crescents are generally associated with severe aggressive disease and occur when there has been a rupture of Bowman's capsule and inflammatory cells have entered the urinary space. An interstitial nephritis affects the interstitium and often the tubules. The vessels are not typically affected. Inflammation of the vessels is termed 'vasculitis'. When acute tubular necrosis has occurred, there are often changes evident on light microscopy.

Answer to Question 46

T, F, F, F, F

Stones tend to lodge in the ureter at the junction of the renal pelvis with the ureter, at the point where the ureter crosses the brim of the bony pelvis and at the junction of the ureter with the bladder. There is typically haematuria, but not proteinuria. Plasma creatinine may rise if a kidney is obstructed but, as the process is usually unilateral, a large rise is seldom seen because the other kidney continues to function normally. Fluids should be encouraged as they will help to move the stone. In addition, dehydration may worsen any renal insult that the obstructed kidney receives. Pain may be referred to the back, the abdomen, the groin and the external genitalia.

Answer to Question 47

1C, 2F, 3G, 4B

There are certain typical presentations of glomerular disease, but it must be remembered that very often the different glomerular pathologies can be difficult to distinguish clinically. For this reason, renal biopsy is extremely useful in clinical practice. Typically, IgA nephropathy can cause recurrent visible haematuria around the time of an upper respiratory tract infection. Minimal change nephropathy is the most common cause of childhood nephrotic syndrome, which is suggested by proteinuria causing frothy urine and swollen ankles. Membranous nephropathy is the most common cause of nephrotic syndrome in adults and often causes renal impairment. In a proportion of cases, it is associated with a malignancy. Goodpasture's disease can cause a rapidly progressive glomerulonephritis which can result in a rapid reduction in urine volume and sometimes even anuria. There is often associated pulmonary haemorrhage causing haemoptysis, because the antiglomerular basement membrane antibodies crossreact with alveolar basement membranes.

Answer to Question 48

F, T, T, F, F

Tuberculosis of the renal and urinary tract, although rare, is well recognized as an important cause of sterile pyuria. If there is any suspicion, repeated urine samples, usually taken in the early morning, should be sent for TB culture, the urinary tract should be imaged and TB should be sought elsewhere in the body. During pregnancy, the ureteric tone is lower and the ureters are more dilated. This makes it easier for infection to ascend to the kidneys. The

common organisms are *Escherichia coli* and *Klebsiella* and *Proteus* species. Superficial *Candida albicans* infection of the perineum is common, but true infection of the urine is not.

Answer to Question 49

1E, 2C, 3B, 4 A

Most cases of what was once termed 'mixed essential cryoglobulinaemia' are now recognized to be caused by hepatitis C virus infection, and may occur with a mesangiocapillary glomerulonephritis. In IgA nephropathy, plasma IgA levels are often raised. Antibodies against double-stranded DNA are typical of SLE. High levels of ANCA and a crescentic glomerulonephritis are typical features of systemic vasculitis such as that of Wegener's granulomatosis. ANCAs are usually antibodies against the contents of neutrophil granules. In Wegener's granulomatosis, the ANCA is typically a cytoplasmic or c-ANCA with specificity against proteinase 3. In microscopic polyangiitis, it is typically a perinuclear or p-ANCA with specificity against myeloperoxidase.

Answer to Question 50

F, F, T, F, F

• Life expectancy of a 40 year old on dialysis is 7–10 years—drastically reduced compared with the general population.

• Carpal tunnel syndrome is usually the result of dialysis-related amyloid which contains β_2-microglobulin

• Homocyst(e)ine levels are substantially elevated compared with the general population, and likely to contribute to the excess cardiovascular risk

• Cholecalciferol (D_3) needs to be hydroxylated by the liver and kidney to $1,25(OH)_2D_3$. Patients with renal impairment should be treated with calcitriol or a vitamin D analogue (e.g. alfacalcidol) that does not require hydroxylation by the kidney

• Haemodialysis patients treated with erythropoietin often become iron deficient.

Answer to Question 51

F, F, F, T, F

Insulin and β-adrenergic agonists stimulate uptake of potassium into cells; calcium has no effect on the potassium level but stabilizes the myocardium. Ion-exchange resins bind and remove potassium via the gastrointestinal tract.

Answer to Question 52

1C, 2E, 3D

Radiocontrast nephropathy typically leads to non-oliguric ARF within 1–3 days of contrast administration; cholesterol embolization can be more progressive, and is associated with evidence of other distal emboli. Pyelonephritis is common in pregnancy and can lead to ARF if there is a solitary kidney.

Answer to Question 53

1F, 2A, 3B, 4B, 5C, 6D, 7F, 8E

• Insulin, simvastatin and alfacalcidol will usually be used in patients with diabetes who have renal impairment. The main side effect of alfacalcidol treatment (used to correct the impaired 1-hydroxylation of cholecalciferol) is hypercalcaemia, and it should be reduced in dose or discontinued if this occurs.

• Glibenclamide is renally excreted, and has a very long half-life in renal impairment. It is best avoided because it can result in prolonged, severe hypoglycaemia. Active metabolites of dextropropoxyphene accumulate in renal impairment, frequently contributing to fatigue, loss of concentration and poor appetite. Metformin is renally excreted and accumulation increases the risk of lactic acidosis.

• Suxamethonium is a depolarizing muscle relaxant (neuromuscular blocking drug) which causes release of potassium from muscle. Lisinopril reduces the amount of aldosterone, thus reducing potassium excretion. Both drugs tend to exacerbate hyperkalaemia.

Answer to Question 54

Diagnoses:
(a) Abdominal aortogram showing renal artery stenosis
(b) CT scan of abdomen showing an adrenal adenoma (Conn's syndrome)
(c) Myxoedematous facies
(d) Retina showing diabetic retinopathy.
Hypertension is likely in (a), (b) and (d).

Answer to Question 55

Non-steroidal anti-inflammatory drugs (NSAIDs) must be used with caution in patients with renal impairment. This is even true of topical preparations, which undergo some systemic absorption. This patient has renal impairment and these drugs could worsen her renal function. Normally, there is tonic prostaglandin-induced renal vasodilatation. NSAIDs inhibit prostaglandin synthesis, thereby inhibiting vasodilatation, which reduces renal blood flow and GFR and promotes renal ischaemia. NSAIDs can also cause interstitial nephritis. In renal disease, other analgesics such as paracetamol should be used where possible. Opiates require care because of accumulation of active metabolites.

The Medical Masterclass series

Clinical Skills

General Clinical Issues

Pain Relief and Palliative Care

Medicine for the Elderly

Emergency Medicine

Infectious Diseases and Dermatology

Infectious Diseases

Dermatology

1 Clinical presentations
  1.1 Blistering disorders
  1.2 Acute generalized rashes
  1.3 Erythroderma
  1.4 A chronic, red facial rash
  1.5 Pruritus
  1.6 Alopecia
  1.7 Abnormal skin pigmentation
  1.8 Patches and plaques on the lower legs
2 Diseases and treatments
  2.1 Alopecia areata
  2.2 Bullous pemphigoid and pemphigoid gestationis
  2.3 Dermatomyositis
  2.4 Mycosis fungoides and Sézary syndrome
  2.5 Dermatitis herpetiformis
  2.6 Drug eruptions
  2.7 Atopic eczema
  2.8 Contact dermatitis
  2.9 Erythema multiforme, Stevens–Johnson syndrome, toxic epidermal necrolysis
  2.10 Erythema nodosum
  2.11 Lichen planus
  2.12 Pemphigus vulgaris
  2.13 Superficial fungal infections
  2.14 Psoriasis
  2.15 Scabies
  2.16 Urticaria and angio-oedema
  2.17 Vitiligo
  2.18 Pyoderma gangrenosum
  2.19 Cutaneous vasculitis
  2.20 Acanthosis nigricans
3 Investigations and practical procedures
  3.1 Skin biopsy
  3.2 Direct and indirect immunofluorescence
  3.3 Patch testing
  3.4 Topical therapy: corticosteroids
  3.5 Phototherapy
  3.6 Systemic retinoids

Haematology and Oncology

Haematology

1 Clinical presentations
  1.1 Microcytic hypochromic anaemia
  1.2 Chest syndrome in sickle cell disease
  1.3 Normocytic anaemia
  1.4 Macrocytic anaemia
  1.5 Hereditary spherocytosis and failure to thrive
  1.6 Neutropenia
  1.7 Pancytopenia
  1.8 Thrombocytopenia and purpura
  1.9 Leucocytosis
  1.10 Lymphocytosis and anaemia
  1.11 Spontaneous bleeding and weight loss
  1.12 Menorrhagia and anaemia
  1.13 Thromboembolism and fetal loss
  1.14 Polycythaemia
  1.15 Bone pain and hypercalcaemia
  1.16 Cervical lymphadenopathy and weight loss
  1.17 Isolated splenomegaly
  1.18 Inflammatory bowel disease with thrombocytosis
  1.19 Transfusion reaction
  1.20 Recurrent deep venous thrombosis
2 Diseases and treatments
  2.1 Causes of anaemia
    2.1.1 Thalassaemia syndromes
    2.1.2 Sickle cell syndromes
    2.1.3 Enzyme defects
    2.1.4 Membrane defects
    2.1.5 Iron metabolism and iron-deficiency anaemia
    2.1.6 Vitamin B_{12} and folate metabolism and deficiency
    2.1.7 Acquired haemolytic anaemia
    2.1.8 Bone-marrow failure and infiltration
  2.2 Haemic malignancy
    2.2.1 Multiple myeloma
    2.2.2 Acute leukaemia—acute lymphoblastic leukaemia and acute myeloid leukaemia
    2.2.3 Chronic lymphocytic leukaemia
    2.2.4 Chronic myeloid leukaemia
    2.2.5 Malignant lymphomas—non-Hodgkin's lymphoma and Hodgkin's disease
    2.2.6 Myelodysplastic syndromes
    2.2.7 Non-leukaemic myeloproliferative disorders
    2.2.8 Amyloidosis
  2.3 Bleeding disorders
    2.3.1 Inherited bleeding disorders
    2.3.2 Acquired bleeding disorders
    2.3.3 Idiopathic thrombocytopenic purpura
  2.4 Thrombotic disorders
    2.4.1 Inherited thrombotic disease
    2.4.2 Acquired thrombotic disease
  2.5 Clinical use of blood products
  2.6 Haematological features of systemic disease
  2.7 Haematology of pregnancy
  2.8 Iron overload
  2.9 Chemotherapy and related therapies
  2.10 Principles of bone-marrow and peripheral blood stem-cell transplantation
3 Investigations and practical procedures
  3.1 The full blood count and film
  3.2 Bone-marrow examination
  3.3 Clotting screen
  3.4 Coombs' test (direct antiglobulin test)
  3.5 Erythrocyte sedimentation rate vs plasma viscosity
  3.6 Therapeutic anticoagulation

Oncology

1 Clinical presentations
  1.1 A lump in the neck
  1.2 Breathlessness and a pelvic mass
  1.3 Breast cancer and headache
    1.3.1 Metastatic disease
  1.4 Cough and weakness
    1.4.1 Paraneoplastic conditions

Cardiology and Respiratory Medicine

Cardiology

Neurology, Ophthalmology and Psychiatry

Neurology

Nephrology

Rheumatology and Clinical Immunology

Index